Hysterectomy

Hysterectomy

edited by

MICHAEL P. DIAMOND MD

Professor, Department of Obstetrics and Gynecology
Director, Division of Reproductive Endocrinology
  and Infertility
Hutzel Hospital, Detroit Medical Center
Wayne State University
Detroit, Michigan

JAMES F. DANIELL MD, FACOG

Clinical Professor, Department of Obstetrics and Gynecology
Vanderbilt University Medical Center
Nashville, Tennessee

HOWARD W. JONES, III MD

Professor, Department of Obstretrics and Gynecology
Director, Gynecologic Oncology
Department of Obstetrics and Gynecology
Vanderbilt University School of Medicine
Nashville, Tennessee

Blackwell Science

Editorial offices:
238 Main Street, Cambridge,
  Massachusetts 02142, USA
Osney Mead, Oxford OX2 0EL, England
25 John Street, London WC1N 2BL,
  England
23 Ainslie Place, Edinburgh EH3 6AJ,
  Scotland
54 University Street, Carlton,
  Victoria 3053, Australia
Arnette Blackwell SA, 1 rue de Lille, 75007
  Paris, France
Blackwell Wissenschafts-Verlag GmbH,
  Kurfürstendamm 57, 10707 Berlin,
  Germany
Blackwell MZV, Feldgasse 13, A-1238
  Vienna, Austria

DISTRIBUTORS:

North America
  Blackwell Science, Inc.
  238 Main Street
  Cambridge, Massachusetts 02142
  (Telephone orders: 800-215-1000 or
                     617-876-7000)

Australia
  Blackwell Science Pty Ltd
  54 University Street
  Carlton, Victoria 3053
  (Telephone orders: 03-347-5552)

Outside North America and Australia
  Blackwell Science, Ltd.
  c/o Marston Book Services, Ltd.
  P.O. Box 87
  Oxford OX2 0DT
  England
  (Telephone orders: 44-865-791155)

Acquisitions: Victoria Reeders
Development: Coleen Traynor
Production: Michelle Choate
Manufacturing: Kathleen Grimes
Typeset by Huron Valley Graphics,
Ann Arbor, MI
Printed and bound by BookCrafters,
Chelsea, MI

© 1995 by Blackwell Science, Inc.

Printed in the United States of America

95 96 97 98 5 4 3 2 1

Notice: The indications and dosages of all
drugs in this book have been recommended
in the medical literature and conform to the
practices of the general medical community.
The medications described do not
necessarily have specific approval by the
Food and Drug Administration for use in
the diseases and dosages for which they are
recommended. The package insert for each
drug should be consulted for use and
dosage as approved by the FDA. Because
standards of usage change, it is advisable to
keep abreast of revised recommendations,
particularly those concerning new drugs.

Library of Congress
Cataloging-in-Publication Data

Hysterectomy / edited by Michael
  Diamond, James F. Daniell, Howard W.
  Jones III.
    p.   cm.
  Includes bibliographical references and
index.
  ISBN 0-86542-255-5
  1. Hysterectomy. 2. Uterus—
Diseases—Treatment. I. Diamond,
Michael P. II. Daniell, James F. III.
Jones, Howard W. (Howard Wilbur),
1942–
  [DNLM: 1. Hysterectomy—
methods. 2. Surgery, Laparoscopic—
methods. 3. Uterine neoplasms—
surgery.   WP 469 H999 1995]
RG391.H9813 1985
818.1'459—dc20
DNLM/DLC
for Library of Congress   94-33710
                                      CIP

Contents

Contributors

JAMES N. ANASTI, *Fellow, National Institutes of Child Health and Human Development, Bethesda, Maryland*

JOEL M. CHILDERS MD, *Clinical Assistant Professor, Division of Gynecologic Oncology, Department of Obstetrics and Gynecology, University of Arizona, Tucson, Arizona*

JAMES F. DANIELL MD, FACOG, *Clinical Professor, Department of Obstetrics and Gynecology, Vanderbilt University Medical Center, Nashville, Tennessee*

ALAN H. DeCHERNEY MD, *Louis E. Phaneuf Professor and Chairman, Department of Obstetrics and Gynecology, Tufts University School of Medicine, Boston, Massachusetts*

MICHAEL P. DIAMOND MD, *Director, Division of Reproductive Endocrinology and Infertility, Professor, Department of Obstetrics and Gynecology, Hutzel Hospital, Detroit Medical Center, Wayne State University, Detroit, Michigan*

ESTHER EISENBERG MD, *Assistant Professor, Vanderbilt University Medical Center, Nashville, Tennessee*

EUGENE F. GUERRE MD, *Clinical Assistant Professor, Department of Obstetrics and Gynecology, Vanderbilt University Medical Center, Nashville, Tennessee*

LARRY DEAN GURLEY MD, *Clinical Instructor, Department of Obstetrics and Gynecology, Vanderbilt Hospital; Director of Laparoscopy Center, Baptist Hospital, Nashville, Tennessee*

JOEL T. HARGROVE MD, *Clinical Professor of Obstetrics and Gynecology, Director of Menopause and PMS Clinics, Vanderbilt University Medical Center; Columbia Menopause Clinic, Columbia, Tennessee*

D. ALAN JOHNS MD, FACOG, *Director, Gynecologic Laparoscopy Center, Harris Methodist Hospital, Fort Worth; Clinical Associate Professor, Department of Obstetrics and Gynecology, University of Texas Southwestern Medical School, Dallas, Texas*

Contributors

HOWARD W. JONES MD, *Professor of Obstetrics and Gynecology, Director of Gynecologic Oncology, Vanderbilt University Medical Center, Nashville, Tennessee*

BRYAN R. KURTZ MD, *Department of Obstetrics and Gynecology, Centennial Medical Center; Clinical Instructor, Department of Obstetrics and Gynecology, Vanderbilt University Medical Center, Nashville, Tennessee*

THOMAS LYONS MD, FACOG, *Athens Women's Clinic, Athens, Georgia*

WILLIAM R. MEYER MD, *Assistant Professor and Director of IVF and Donor Gametes Program, Division of Reproductive Endocrinology, Department of Obstetrics and Gynecology, University of North Carolina at Chapel Hill, Chapel Hill, North Carolina*

KEVIN G. OSTEEN PhD, *Associate Professor of Obstetrics and Gynecology, Vanderbilt University Medical Center, Nashville, Tennessee*

ALAN S. PENZIAS MD, *Assistant Professor, Department of Obstetrics and Gynecology, Tufts University School of Medicine, Boston, Massachusetts*

GUY J. PHOTOPULOS MD, *Associate Professor and Director, Division of Gynecologic Oncology, Department of Obstetrics and Gynecology, University of Tennessee, Memphis, Tennessee*

DEIRDRE ROBINSON MD, *Assistant Professor, Section on Gynecology, Bowman Gray School of Medicine of Wake Forest University, Winston-Salem, North Carolina*

LESLIE A. SHARP MD, FACOG, *Clinical Associate Professor of Obstetrics and Gynecology, University of Minnesota; Director, Fairview Endosurgery Center, Minneapolis, Minnesota*

THOMAS G. STOVALL MD, *Associate Professor and Head, Section On Gynecology, Bowman Gray School of Medicine of Wake Forest University, Winston-Salem, North Carolina*

LAURA WILLIAMS MD, *Clinical Assistant Professor of Gynecologic Oncology, Vanderbilt University Medical Center, Nashville, Tennessee*

Hysterectomy

1 Hysterectomy: An Introduction

MICHAEL P. DIAMOND & JAMES F. DANIELL

Hysterectomy. A simple concept, yet a procedure that has various physical, psychological, and emotional implications for the women that undergo the procedure. For some, it means an end to catamenial pain and inconveniences; for others it represents an abrupt, unwanted termination of the potential for spontaneous procreation.

In 1980, hysterectomy was the most common major operative procedure performed in women. The most common indications include uterine fibroids, dysfunctional uterine bleeding, adenomyosis, and pelvic pain, as well as malignancies of the uterine fundus and cervix. However, with the exception of the latter indication, the appropriate timing of hysterectomy may often be quite variable and controversial. For example, no definitive consensus exists as to the extent to which conservative methods of management, e.g., hormonal regulation for dysfunctional uterine bleeding (DUB), should continue before progressing to operative intervention. Twenty-five percent of all hysterectomies are performed for DUB, and if properly screened and counseled, many of those patients could be potentially managed with ablation of the endometrium via hysteroscopy. This emerging alternative to hysterectomies for the group of symptomatic patients with DUB is the most minimally invasive of surgical procedures; however, the long-term efficacy of this procedure remains to be fully determined. Additionally, variation exists concerning the threshold for operative intervention for subjective symptoms such as pelvic pain. For the most part, this diversity in hysterectomy indications is probably directly responsible for the difference in the rates of hysterectomy procedures in different regions of the United States.

Traditionally, hysterectomies were performed by both abdominal and vaginal routes. Comparisons of complications of these two approaches have generally yielded various rates of morbidity. Postoperative infections in the antibiotic era are greatly reduced from years ago and are currently estimated to be 58% for vaginal procedures and 36% for abdominal procedures (1). However, the need for blood transfusions as a sequela of hemorrhage occurred in 8% of vaginal hysterectomies and 15% of abdominal hysterectomies, and overall complication rates were 25% and 43%, respectively (1). Additionally, it is generally considered that the length of hospital stay and the time to recovery are shorter with vaginal hysterectomies (1–3).

[1]

NEXT PARA RESET

Interestingly, despite the overall reduced risk of complications and the decreased morbidity associated with hysterectomies performed by a vaginal approach, most hysterectomies performed in the United States utilize an abdominal approach (2,4,5). The explanation(s) for this paradox is unclear, but may represent insufficient training in vaginal surgery during obstetrical and gynecological residencies, reflected by subsequent limited performance of vaginal procedures.

Alternatively, the relatively high frequency of abdominal hysterectomies may reflect the large number and diversity of relative contraindications to vaginal hysterectomy that have been described (Table 1-1). Importantly, the extent of pathology required to cause a vaginal procedure to be contraindicated may vary greatly with the training and experience of the surgeon. For example, some vaginal surgeons would consider a 12- to 14-week-sized uterus too large to remove vaginally; others would set this limit at a 16- to 18-week-sized uterus.

For many of the relative contraindications to vaginal hysterectomy, concomitant laparoscopy may be of value, by allowing conversion of what would have been an abdominal hysterectomy to one performed vaginally. For patients with pelvic pain, performance of a diagnostic laparoscopy identifies the presence of pelvic pathology. Therapy is then initiated by laparotomy, vaginally, or laparoscopically. For patients with no intra-abdominal pathology, vaginal hysterectomy is suggested. Alternatively, some women found to have adhesions, endometriosis, adnexal masses, and other indications can then be treated by one of the three means of entry into the abdominal cavity. Highly experienced vaginal surgeons may choose to treat abdominal pathology vaginally; individuals well trained in endoscopic surgery can intervene therapeutically by laparoscopy, thus avoiding the necessity of laparotomy. (Of course, relative efficacy of procedures performed abdominally, vaginally, or laparoscopically has been rarely assessed in well-designed studies. Thus "the best" approach is unfortunately determined by anecdotal experiences of individual surgeons rather than by clinical trials.) This combination of laparoscopic surgery followed by completion of the operative procedure vaginally, is known as laparoscopically assisted vaginal hysterectomy (LAVH).

Unfortunately, the reports to date that have described "LAVH" represent the widely discrepant extent of the endoscopic portion of the surgical procedure. These range from diagnostic laparoscopy followed

Table 1-1 Contraindications to vaginal hysterectomy described in the gynecological literature

Excessive uterine enlargement
Adnexal masses
Pelvic pain
History of abdominal surgery
History or suspicion of endometriosis
History or suspicion of pelvic adhesions
History or suspicion of pelvic inflammatory disease
Nulliparity
Lack of uterine descensus
Unexplained pelvic pain

Stage

0—Laparoscopy done—No laparoscopic procedure performed prior to vaginal hysterectomy
1—Procedure included laparoscopic adhesiolysis and/or excision of endometriosis
2—Either or both adnexa freed laparoscopically
3—Bladder dissected from uterus
4—Uterine artery transected laparoscopically
5—Anterior and/or posterior colpotomy or entire uterus freed
SUBSCRIPT—
    0—Neither ovary excised
    1—One ovary excised
    2—Both ovaries excised

NOTE—If the extent of the procedure performed laparoscopically varied on the right and left pelvic sidewalls, stage the procedure by the most advanced side. (Reproduced with permission from Johns DA, Diamond MP. Laparoscopically assisted vaginal hysterectomies. J Reprod Med 1994;39:424–428.)

by total vaginal hysterectomy to a complete laparoscopic hysterectomy, including total laparoscopic uterine excision and vaginal vault closure. Such extensive diversity makes even descriptive comparison of LAVH difficult to interpret. To allow more objective comparison of LAVH procedures, Johns and Diamond (6) developed an LAVH classification system (Table 1-2).

A controversial variation of LAVH gaining popularity both in the U.S. and abroad that we will discuss in Chapter 7 is the laparoscopic subtotal or supracervical hysterectomy (LSH). Proponents of LSH suggest that avoiding laparoscopic dissection around the cervix removes the risks of ureteral and bladder injuries, retains the body of the cervix to reduce risks of later vault prolapse, and may lessen the chances of cuff injections. The body of the uterus may be removed via colpotomy, morcellation, or enlarging the umbilical laparoscopic incision. A combination excisional cervical cone may be used to prophylactically reduce the central squamous columnar cervical cells, while leaving the lateral fibromuscular cervix for support. Long-term outcome following this procedure remains to be fully documented.

There are several major concerns regarding the performance of LAVH. One is the cost of the procedure. Laparoscopic surgical procedures have generally been considered to save money. However, this may represent a "false economy." Early reports describing cost savings of laparoscopic procedures primarily represented a savings attributable to a decreased length of hospital stay rather than a reduction in operating room expenses. Differences in length of hospitalization, however, may, in large part, be based upon physician preconceptions on how long patients should remain hospitalized postoperatively. For example, years ago, pregnant women often remained hospitalized after a delivery for a week or more; now postpartum hospitalization is considerably shorter. Similarly, the recently held preconceptions that women undergoing abdominal hysterectomy should remain until the fifth or sixth postoperative day and women undergoing vaginal hysterectomy need to remain until the

[3]

third or fourth postoperative day need reappraisal. This length of hospitalization will frequently not be necessary. Because of their preconceptions, physicians often inform patients of these routine lengths of hospitalization. Consequently, the patients may now expect hospitalization for a longer time and may, therefore, be content to remain for the duration. Giving patients different expectations, as is done with LAVH, when patients are often told to expect to go home either the same day as the operation or no later than the second postoperative day, will often result in earlier hospital discharges with resultant cost savings. Armed with the information that LAVH patients have been able to be discharged sooner after a major operative procedure,—in conjunction with revised physician and patient expectations—patients who undergo abdominal or vaginal hysterectomies are now often going home sooner.

It should be noted that the earlier anticipated discharge may in part be self-fulfilling because of changes in care practice. These changes may include differences in preoperative premedication, choice of alternative anesthetic agents and/or dosage, earlier postoperative ambulation, and more postoperative liberalized diet advancement.

Another area of discussion with regard to cost is the use of disposable instrumentation. Use of disposable instruments has markedly increased during the last five years. Advocates claim the advantages are increased safety, sharpness, sterility, and rapid availability. The questions, however, are whether these theoretical advantages are real and cost-effective. The expense issue of these instruments is further compounded by the hospitals that frequently charge the patient double or triple the original price.

A second area of extensive discussion regarding LAVH is who can perform the procedure, specifically, what should be required to learn how to perform the procedures. Related questions are how many cases must be performed prior to developing sufficient expertise to allow unsupervised performance of LAVH, who should credential surgeons, and whether recertification should be required. Additionally, some claim that LAVH should be considered an experimental procedure conducted only under the auspices of an institutional review board-approved protocol. Unfortunately, there is much disagreement on these issues, leaving the answers extremely unclear. The issue is further clouded by other factors: the competition between different surgeons and their hospitals for patients, difficulty of being the first in a community to acquire expertise, limitations of surgeons gaining hands-on experience away from their own institutions, and medicolegal issues involved with "certifying" another physician (or failing to do so). These issues are not specific to LAVH but extend to other forms of advanced endoscopic procedures as well. Furthermore, many would claim that these issues are relevant for procedures also performed by laparotomy or vaginally.

Safety of LAVH represents a third issue of concern. Currently, studies describing the performance of, and complications associated with, LAVH are limited. Additionally, the current series that do exist have been primarily performed by extremely experienced endoscopic surgeons. The extent to which the frequency and type of complications

[4]

experienced by this select group of physicians can be extended to other, less experienced surgeons is unclear but will probably represent an underestimation of the complications that are likely to occur.

Lastly, a great deal of controversy exists with regard to the need for procedures that replace abdominal or vaginal hysterectomy and what should be required to establish equivalent or improved efficacy compared to those more traditional approaches.

It is with these issues in mind that the need for this book was conceived. The hope is to present the traditional forms of hysterectomy, with indications, contraindications, complications, and considerations, and to have these serve as the background upon which the newer endoscopic techniques can be judged. These new alternatives include more conservative treatments of uterine pathology as well as laparoscopic approaches to hysterectomy.

References

1 Burnett LS. Gynecologic history, examination, and operations. In: Jones HW III, Wentz AC, Burnett LS, eds. Novak's textbook of gynecology, 11th edition. Williams and Wilkins, Baltimore, 1988:3–39.

2 Dicker RC, Greenspan JR, Strauss LT, et al. Complications of abdominal and vaginal hysterectomy among women of reproductive age in the United States. The Collaborative review of sterilization. Am J Obstet Gynecol 1982;144:841–848.

3 White SC, Wartel LJ, Wade ME. Comparison of abdominal and vaginal hysterectomies. Obstet Gynecol 1971;37:530–537.

4 Dicker RC, Scally MJ, Greenspan JR, et al. Hysterectomy among women of reproductive age: trends in the United States, 1970–1978. JAMA, 1982:248:323–327.

5 Kovac SR, Cruikshank SH, Retto HF. Laparoscopy-assisted vaginal hysterectomy. J Gyn Surg 1990;6:185.

6 Johns DA, Diamond MP. Laparoscopically assisted vaginal hysterectomies. J Reprod Med 1994;39:424–428.

2 Hysterectomy: Abdominal Approach

WILLIAM R. MEYER & JAMES N. ANASTI

The removal of the uterus abdominally may be an evanescent art. One must wonder whether the most frequently performed operation, second only to cesarean section, will be forgotten and condemned as obsolete. This may occur as familiarity with medical and surgical alternatives to total abdominal hysterectomy (TAH) increases. As a result, a discussion and, at times, possibly even a defense of the procedure of abdominal hysterectomy in our current era of advanced operative endoscopy seems appropriate. Accordingly, a review of the indications for abdominal hysterectomy past and present along with key operative techniques will be presented. Current alternatives to abdominal hysterectomy will be considered. A section on the difficult aspects of abdominal hysterectomy will complete the chapter.

Abdominal hysterectomy

In 1986, the first members of the "baby boom" era turned 40, so, based on age alone, the heart of this population is at greatest risk for hysterectomy for the next 10 to 15 years (Table 2-1). Accordingly, the absolute number of hysterectomies is estimated to rise from the approximately 670,000 in 1985 to 810,000 in 1995 and finally to 854,000 in 2005 unless modifications in the need for hysterectomy occur (1). In the United States, about one in every three women have undergone a hysterectomy by age 60, reflecting a national rate that is twice that seen in many Western European countries (2). A recent study involving 12,000 women in 15 states and the District of Columbia showed that women with less education and lower incomes are more likely to undergo hysterectomy (3). These numbers, especially those representing socioeconomic strata, continue to elicit concern regarding procedural necessity, especially as the field of gynecology becomes more competitive and the need to demonstrate advanced operative skill at laparoscopy, including laparoscopic hysterectomy, increases. The path for unnecessary hysterectomy may widen.

Unfortunately, the empiric use of the phrase "unnecessary surgery" has no value unless adequately defined. Its definition is obviously difficult. In an attempt to clarify this term, hospital quality assurance pro-

Table 2-1 Rate of hysterectomies for all females and for females with intact uteri by age: United States, 1984

Age (years)	All females	Females with intact uteri
15–19	0.1[a]	0.1[a]
20–24	1.7	1.7
25–29	6.1	6.3
30–34	9.3	9.9
35–39	14.7	17.1
40–44	16.2	20.3
45–49	15.8	23.0
50–54	7.8	11.8
55–59	4.3	6.8
60–64	4.4	7.0
65–69	4.8	7.2
70–74	4.4	6.9
75–79	3.1	5.0
80–84	2.5	4.3
85 ≥	0.5[a]	1.0[a]
Total 15 years ≥	6.9	8.6

[a]Estimates based on cell size less than 30 cases.
National Center for Health Statistics. Hysterectomies in the United States 1965–1984. National Health Survey Series 13. No. 92. Maryland: DNNS Publication No. (PNS) 1987, 87-1753.

grams and insurance companies have used various methods to lessen the public's perception of the abundance of unindicated surgery. One simple solution proposed has been the need for the second operative opinion. McCarthy and Kamons reported that nearly 43.9% of the cases scheduled for hysterectomy and reviewed by a second consulting physician were unconfirmed for surgery (4). However, in a more contemporary review of 1698 women required to obtain a second opinion prior to undergoing hysterectomy, only 8% of these cases were felt to be unjustified (5). In this last study, even the patients themselves may have contributed independently to the number of unindicated hysterectomies. For example, women in the South and North Central regions of the country tended to undergo surgery even when unconfirmed preoperatively by the consulting physician or postoperatively by defined pathology.

Obviously, the use of second opinion will not completely restrict the performance of unindicated hysterectomy. Although designed to pass cost savings on to third party payers, the value of second opinion programs may be more toward improved patient education, improved health care, and enhanced communication between physician and patient. Although these intangible benefits may exist, perceived monetary savings have prompted both Medicare and Medicaid programs to require a second opinion prior to hysterectomy.

Reiter and Gambone have noted that the so-called inappropriate hysterectomy may be more commonly associated with the gynecologist's liberal use of multiple preoperative indications for surgery (6). In fact, these same authors have reported a 24% reduction in the number of hysterectomies performed when the surgeon was required to select a single preoperative indication from a predetermined list (7). Their report supports Thompson and Birch's contention that surgery is no more justified if the surgeon compiles a complex list of inappropriate or partially indicated reasons for hysterectomy when one solid indication cannot be supported (8).

Despite efforts to limit the number of preoperative indications, the increased demand for operative laparoscopic procedures with reduced convalescence may lead both physician and patient alike to consent to surgery with even more nebulous preoperative justifications. Soon the postoperative standardized list delineating justifiable indications for hysterectomy rather than a postoperative perfunctory review by the hospital tissue review committee may become a prerequisite.

Indications

Excluding gynecologic malignancy, Thompson and Birch listed the indications for hysterectomy and specified those cases in which an abdominal approach was considered more appropriate than a vaginal one (3). This list included leiomyomatous uterus, ectopic pregnancy, endometriosis, obstetrical catastrophes, chronic pelvic pain, and recurrent dysfunctional uterine bleeding. A decade later, many of these recommendations remain pertinent while others have been modified by newer medicinal and surgical management.

Leiomyomatous uterus

The most common reason for performing a hysterectomy is the presence of leiomyomas (1,9). Although often clinically occult, 77% of women undergoing hysterectomy will be found to have myomas (10). The clinical incidence of myomata that necessitates treatment reaches a peak at age 45 (Table 2-2).

Table 2-2 Annual rate of hysterectomy for myomas and endometriosis (1982–1984) (Rate per 1000 females with intact uteri per year)

Age group	Myoma	Endometriosis
15–24	0.02	0.14
25–34	1.16	2.26
35–44	7.29	4.56
45–54	7.74	2.61
55–64	0.63	0.17
> 65	0.36	0.06

National Center for Health Statistics. Hysterectomies in the United States 1965–1984. National Health Survey Series 13. No. 92. Maryland: DHHS Publication No. (PNS) 1987, 87-1753.

Symptomatic leiomyomas are usually associated with dyspareunia, dysmenorrhea, menometrorrhagia, and/or urinary frequency, prompting uterine removal. Risk factors for myomas, other than age, seem to correlate best with the "unopposed estrogen" model used to explain the etiology of endometrial and breast cancer along with endometriosis (11). Thus, higher parity, leanness, smoking, and exercise may lower the incidence of myomas. Interestingly, a protective effect has been noted with oral contraceptive use (12). Even in asymptomatic cases, abdominal hysterectomy for a uterus of greater than 12 weeks' size has long been recommended by the American College of Obstetricians and Gynecologists based on uterine size alone (13), although this also is coming into question. The main justification being that an enlarged, leiomyomatous uterus lends interference to bimanual palpation and clinical evaluation of adnexae. Presently, the combination of tumor markers and transvaginal sonography may allow the clinician adequate evaluation of the adnexae, obviating the previous indications for abdominal hysterectomy (14). Unfortunately, one of the most common serum tumor markers used for detection of ovarian cancer, CA-125, may also be elevated in myomatous disease. Similar to patients with endometriosis, women with ovarian cancer have mean CA-125 levels several-fold higher than women with fibroids (15). In difficult sonographic cases, magnetic resonance may assist in distinguishing myomas from ovarian malignancies. The latter demonstrates a high signal on T-2-weighted images (16).

Other investigators have recommended prophylactic hysterectomy in asymptomatic women with smaller myomatous uteri due to a perceived increased morbidity associated with hysterectomy for leiomyomas in women with uteri greater than 12 weeks' size. Reiter et al. evaluated this theory in 93 women with leiomyomata of various sizes. Women with enlarged uteri were no more likely to suffer perioperative complications, including blood loss, than were women with smaller uteri (17). This study, however, should not be taken as evidence to discount the beneficial effects that gonadotropin-releasing hormonal (GnRH) agonists have on diminishing uterine volume in myomatous disease. In these cases, GnRH agonists have been noted not only to decrease fibroid size but also to decrease surrounding myometrial tissue size, with a resultant decrease in uterine vascular perfusion as measured by Doppler flow (18,19). Lumsden et al. divided a group of 27 patients with myomas undergoing hysterectomy into no preoperative medical treatment versus three months of GnRH agonist therapy. A significant decrease in blood loss was noted in the GnRH agonist-treated group (350 ml vs 235 ml, $p < 0.01$) (20). In these cases, reduction of surgical morbidity is the goal. Other potential advantages from GnRH prehysterectomy treatment may include decreased risk of urologic injury, performance of Pfannenstiel's incision, and increased preoperative hemoglobin concentrations prior to surgery.

GnRH agonists have also been effectively used in a study in which 76% of women with 14- to 18-week-size myomatous uteri underwent successful vaginal hysterectomy after medical therapy (21). Additionally, perimenopausal women with symptomatic fibroids may use GnRH ago-

[9]

nists successfully to induce a hypoestrogenic milieu, and, once the patients are asymptomatic, hormonal add-back therapy may be considered. Sequential add-back therapy after a three-month GnRH-agonist-only period is more successful than simultaneous GnRH-estrogen-progestin administration in attaining adequate uterine volume reduction. It seems that 0.3 mg of conjugated equine estrogens in add-back therapy is inadequate to prevent hypoestrogenic symptoms. In sequential add-back therapy, cardioprotective as well as osteoconservative estrogen therapy may be reinstituted without persistent uterine size reduction (22). Interestingly, gestrinone (ethinyl-nor-testosterone derivative), which has both antiestrogen and antiprogesterone effects, has caused 40% maximal uterine volume shrinkage with a year of therapy (23). In contrast to GnRH analogue therapy, uterine regrowth is slow with gestrinone (24). Obviously, these generalized cases illustrate that the absolute need for hysterectomy, especially transabdominally, can no longer be recommended based solely on the size of the leiomyomatous uterus.

An enlarging uterus during GnRH agonist therapy must alert the clinician to the suspicion of leiomyosarcoma. The latter produces symptoms similar to those induced by myomas. Anecdotal reports of unsuspected non-enlarging leiomyosarcomas discovered at the time of myomectomy or hysterectomy in perimenopausal women pretreated with GnRH agonists have been reported (25,26). These cases illustrate GnRH agonists' limited use as the panacea for avoidance of surgical intervention in myomatous disease, especially in this age group.

Ectopic pregnancy

Rarely is hysterectomy indicated in cases involving an ectopic gestation. In women with severe tubal disease secondary to repetitive tubal ectopic pregnancies, uterine conservation is recommended as in vitro fertilization offers an increasingly more successful means of attaining an intrauterine pregnancy. The treatment of cervical ectopic pregnancies, however, has routinely been surgical—requiring abdominal hysterectomy in approximately 50% of cases (Figure 2-1). Certain conservative measures have been attempted in the treatment of cervical ectopic pregnancies. These measures have included bilateral hypogastric artery ligation,

Figure 2-1 Decade by decade breakdown of total number of reported cervical ectopic pregnancies, number treated with hysterectomy, and number resulting in death.

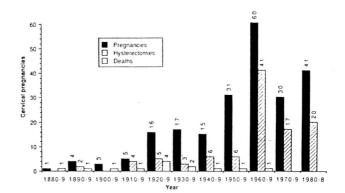

removal of the conception and cervical packing; cervical cerclage prior to evacuation; Foley catheter tamponade of the cervix; and uterine artery embolization (27). Unfortunately, in most cases, profuse hemorrhage is often the result, necessitating emergent abdominal hysterectomy. Recently, the use of chemotherapy, specifically methotrexate, has modified the approach to ectopic gestation. Farabow et al. were the first to attempt to treat, albeit unsuccessfully, a cervical pregnancy in 1983 with methotrexate (28). Others have used methotrexate successfully to conservatively treat cervical pregnancies (29,30).

Similar to Yankowitz et al., our illustrative case demonstrates that a single intramuscular injection of methotrexate (50 mg/M2), may allow evacuation of a cervical pregnancy with uterine conservation (29). Theoretically, this drug may limit peritrophoblastic vascularity, allowing curettage with reduced blood loss (Figure 2-2). Again, an absolute indication for abdominal hysterectomy becomes obsolete, especially when fertility conservation may be desirable.

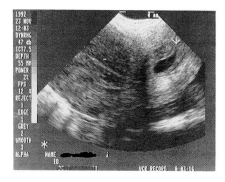

Figure 2-2 Cervical ectopic pregnancy detected by transvaginal sonography.

Endometriosis

Despite relatively new medical modalities and conservative surgery, recurrence of endometriosis is a frequent problem. Medical therapy is often unsuccessful due to intolerance of androgenic or hypoestrogenic effects of danocrine or GnRH agonists, respectively.

Laparoscopy may be unsuccessful in long-term eradication of the disease due to the inability of the surgeon to appreciate subperitoneal and subserosal endometrial implants, ovarian endometriomas, or limited long-term data on more radical laparoscopic surgery, including bilateral oophorectomy. In fact, subsequent reoperations for endometriosis in women treated by a conservative operative approach, with or without medical therapy, has varied 2–47% (31,32,33).

Presently, the only definitive treatment for endometriosis is hysterectomy and bilateral oophorectomy. The most dramatic increase in the hysterectomy rate has been confined to cases specifically performed for endometriosis. From 1965–1967 to 1982–1984, the rate of hysterectomy for endometriosis has increased 2.2-fold (1). Should endometriosis occur based on Sampson's implantation theory, then hysterectomy removes the primary source of ectopic implants (34). Although hysterectomy may eliminate endometriosis-associated dysmenorrhea, chronic pelvic pain may recur or persist. When a semiconservative operation (hysterectomy only) is performed, studies indicate a 0–6% incidence of reoperation due to endometriosis (35,36). The incidence of reoperation for recurrent endometriosis after definitive treatment, including hysterectomy and castration, is much lower, between 0 and 2.5%, as reported in two large studies (37,38). However, radical surgery is not without its shortcomings as re-exploration may be necessary for ovarian remnant tissue (39). In these cases, either functioning remnant ovarian tissue or its reactivation of residual endometriosis may be problematic to the woman. Ovarian remnant tissue should be suspected with cyclic pain and borderline gonadotropin levels. Although these symptoms need not exist to suspect the disease, ovarian exogenous stimulation with either clomiphene citrate or gonadotropins may help delineate remnant tissue sonographically (40).

The use of hormonal therapy after abdominal hysterectomy and bilateral salpingo-oophorectomy for endometriosis remains controversial. The low incidence of reactivation of endometriosis, reported from 0 to 3.9%, allows one to use estrogen replacement safely (41,42). It is important to remove evidence of infiltrative intestinal disease, as this may be re-exacerbated during hormonal replacement therapy.

As can be seen, abdominal hysterectomy remains a viable option for the treatment of severe endometriosis. The use of bilateral oophorectomy should be recommended in those cases in which childbearing is complete and severe disease remains or, possibly, in cases of severe pelvic pain in which infiltrating bowel lesions are present. If the bowel lesion is extensive, reducing the lumen, resection of the bowel is indicated regardless of patient age (43).

Peripartum

In discussing nebulous preoperative indications for hysterectomy, one is reminded of the more obvious cases. These would include the emergent abdominal hysterectomy performed in order to preserve a mother's life due to intractable uterine bleeding in the peripartum period.

Peripartum hysterectomy may include the elective cesarean hysterectomy, the emergent cesarean hysterectomy, or the emergent postpartum hysterectomy. Elective cesarean hysterectomy for the purpose of sterilization has been replaced by cesarean section and tubal ligation or postpartum mini-laparotomy sterilization once the risk of perinatal infant mortality has lessened.

Chestnut et al. have used elective cesarean hysterectomy when sterilization was accompanied by other gynecologic maladies, including cervical intraepithelial neoplasia, microinvasive cervical cancer, multiple or degenerating leiomyomata, chronic pelvic inflammatory disease, and menstrual aberrations (44). Surprisingly, this approach may be preferable, as a recent study demonstrates that the operative morbidity of elective cesarean hysterectomy versus cesarean section followed by an abdominal hysterectomy within several years is unchanged (45). Emergent peripartum cesarean hysterectomy is most commonly performed for uterine rupture, uterine atony, and placental abnormalities, such as accreta or previa (46). Chorioamnionitis with sepsis may also dictate cesarean hysterectomy (Table 2-3). Of course, certain obstetrical scenarios should alert the physician to the increased possibility of peripartum hysterectomy. These include delivery in a grand multiparous woman or previous cesarean section in a woman with a presently suspected low-lying anterior placenta or placenta previa. Unique operative technical problems in cesarean hysterectomy will be discussed under techniques of abdominal hysterectomy.

[12]

Table 2-3 Cesarean hysterectomy indications

Emergent	Percent	Indicated nonemergent	Percent	Elective	Percent
Placenta accreta	5	Fibroids	13	Repeat C/S ($\geq$ 3)	30
previa	4	Cervical neoplasia	10	C/S and sterilization	10
abruptio (pph)	11	Repeat C/S, defective scar	8	Grand multiparity and sterilization	7
Uterine rupture	7	Chorioamnionitis, sepsis	6		
Uterine atony (pph)	5				
Uterine artery laceration (C/S)	3				
TOTALS:	26		37		47

pph (postpartum hemorrhage)
C/S (cesarean section)
Modified from Plauche WC. Cesarean hysterectomy: indications, technique, and complications. In: Pitkin RM, Scott JR, eds. Clinical obstetrics and gynecology. J.B. Lippincott Co, 1986;29:318–328.

Chronic pelvic pain

It is estimated that 10 to 13% of all hysterectomies are done for chronic pelvic pain, or pain that has persisted for at least six months (47,48). New theories concerning the understanding of pelvic pain transmission have recently emerged. The gate theory allows for modulation of peripheral nociceptive signals by motivational and affective control. Therefore, chronic pelvic pain may lead to depression that may intensify the perception of pelvic pain by opening this gate, allowing more nociceptive signals to pass to the brain (49). Thus, mood and pain become more intermingled. This may explain why half of the women with chronic pelvic pain and negative laparoscopy have either psychogenic pain or a demonstrable somatization disorder (50,51). Due to this last observation, attempts at nonsurgical management of chronic pelvic pain have been intensified. Classically, operative intervention is delayed until most nonsurgical avenues have been pursued (52).

Nonextirpative operative management of pelvic pain may include diagnostic laparoscopy, lysis of adhesions, exfulguration of endometriosis, uterosacral nerve ablation, and presacral neurectomy. Abdominal hysterectomy for pelvic pain may be most clearly indicated in cases of leiomyomata or adenomyosis. The latter case may be effectively diagnosed preoperatively with magnetic resonance (53).

A recent study evaluated a long-term follow-up of women who underwent hysterectomy for chronic pelvic pain (nonadnexal) thought to be uterine in origin. Nearly a quarter of the 99 women studied continued to have pelvic pain postoperatively. Interestingly, over a third of the cases treated with vaginal hysterectomy had persistent pain. This study demonstrates that hysterectomy may be effective treatment for pelvic pain in most women (54). However, vaginal hysterectomy without at least initial laparoscopic surveillance and evaluation cannot be recommended for the treatment of pelvic pain—even when that pain is thought to be of uterine origin.

[13]

Preoperative considerations

As discussed, the necessity to perform an abdominal hysterectomy is rarely emergent. Adequate time should be set aside for preoperative counseling of the patient as well as a discussion with her and her family about the risks, benefits, side effects, and alternatives to abdominal hysterectomy. Concerns about blood transfusions, posthysterectomy sexuality, and ovarian conservation should be addressed at this time. Because of the inquisitive and, unfortunately, litigious nature of our society, an illustrated anatomical text such as Netter's *The CIBA Collection of Medical Illustrations: Reproductive System* on pelvic anatomy is useful, allowing the patient to visualize her anatomy and also to delineate the organs to be removed. Written chart documentation of this particular step is suggested.

As alluded to, patients' concerns about the need for blood may be ameliorated by autologous donation or use of the cell saver in non-infected or noncontaminated, noncancerous conditions. One unit of autologous blood may be donated every 72 hours as long as the patient continues oral iron supplements and her hematocrit remains above 33%. Autologous units may be stored 5–6 weeks (55).

Autologous donors should be questioned about any bouts of diarrhea at the time of donation up to the anticipated day of surgery. Autologous transfusions of this blood, potentially contaminated with enteric bacteria, have been blamed for severe autotransfusion reactions (56). Various women's support groups, including HERS (Hysterectomy Educational Resources & Services, Philadelphia, PA), provide educational programs for women contemplating hysterectomy. This group's literature has described a "posthysterectomy syndrome" in at least 35% of women undergoing hysterectomy *without* removal of the ovaries (57,58). Supposed symptoms of posthysterectomy syndrome include hot flashes, loss of libido, memory loss, insomnia, and vaginal atrophy (59). Others may concur with the theory of decreased sexual response after hysterectomy, while still others dispute these findings (60).

Perioperative considerations

Skin preparation

The skin represents the patient's initial line of defense against infection. Unfortunately, the amount of operating room time and money spent on skin preparation exceeds its contribution toward reducing wound infection. The use of a preoperative bath is not warranted unless skin colonization with *Staphyloccocus aureus* is known (61). The specific agent used in the preparation of the skin is also of little importance. Application of the antimicrobial agent by painting or spraying is as effective as the time-honored, traditionally used, long mechanical scrub. In addition, vaginal irrigation with a saline solution is as effective as povidone-iodine use in the setting of vaginal hysterectomy with prophylactic antibiotic use (62). Others have found that preoperative vaginal and perineal scrubbing 12 hours prior to surgery, along with a vaginal tampon soaked in iodine and left in place until surgery, was as effective as perioperative ampicillin in reducing postoperative infectious morbidity (63). The ever-increasing incidence of pseudomembranous colitis makes alternatives to antibiotic use worth considering. Compared to skin preparation, hair removal is an important issue in infection rates. Shaving hair with a razor increases wound infection rates, while clipping or trimming hair in the operating room is acceptable (64,65).

Prophylactic antibiotic use

While perioperative prophylactic antibiotic use at the time of vaginal hysterectomy in premenopausal women is unquestionably effective, the benefit at the time of abdominal hysterectomy is more controversial (66,67). Unfortunately, distinctions between wound infection, cuff abscess, pelvic cellulitis, and urinary tract infections are not always separately delineated in studies evaluating chemoprophylaxis in the scenario of abdominal hysterectomy. Houang, in an excellent review on the subject, suggested that double-blind placebo control studies should be made within each gynecologic institute of practice prior to the decision on a set individual policy of prophylactic antibiotic use (68). Thompson echoes this dictum when he states that perioperative prophylactic antibiotic use in abdominal hysterectomy should "not be used routinely unless the patient population served has an inherently high risk of postoperative sepsis. Of course, perioperative antibiotics should be used on an individual basis when there is evidence of interference with natural host defenses in any patient" (69).

The use of an extensive mechanical bowel preparation with electrolytic osmotic solutions and antibiotics is excessive unless bowel involvement by endometriosis, cancer, or extensive pelvic adhesions is suspected. In these cases, a 3-day preparation is preferred over the 1-day. Laxatives and clear liquids are begun on the first day. Nightly tap water enemas are given. Erythromycin (1 g) and neomycin (1 g) are given four times daily during the 48 hours prior to surgery (70). In a "routine" abdominal hysterectomy, a clear liquid diet the day before surgery, with enemas until clear the night prior to and the morning of surgery, is sufficient.

Operative technique

Positioning

Patient positioning, often dismissed as trivial, may facilitate the operation from beginning to end, including the examination under anesthesia to the posthysterectomy cystoscopy.

Positioning is begun after anesthesia is administered. The patient's legs are placed in the Allen universal stirrups, hips flexed approximately 15° on the horizontal. The weight of the legs should fall not on the calf, but on the heel of the foot, decreasing potential venous congestion. This

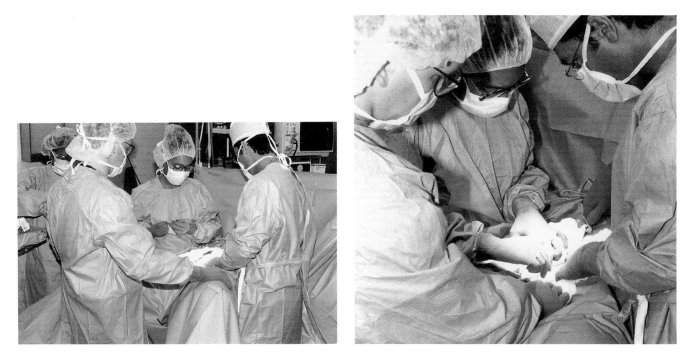

Figure 2-3 Patient positioning allows for better operative assistance and optimal visualization and exposure.

positioning is also felt to decrease strain on the lumbar spine (Figure 2-3). This manner of positioning allows several other advantages than those mentioned above. These advantages include access to the anterior vaginal wall for suprapubic colpourethropexy along with second assistant positioning between the legs for more optimal visualization and exposure. This positioning also allows one to place a sponge stick forcep in the posterior fornix to delineate upper vaginal limits during rectovaginal dissection in cases of endometriosis or severe pelvic adhesive disease. The exam is performed under anaesthesia after a Foley catheter is placed in the bladder for continuous drainage. This exam may cause the surgeon to modify his or her original surgical approach, beginning with the incision.

Incision

The incision determines access to the pelvis. A common dictum is not to forfeit exposure for cosmetic results. Many benign gynecological procedures can be performed through a Pfannenstiel incision. Yet, when cases involve a large leiomyomatous uterus, extensive adhesions, or severe endometriosis in which the abdominal over the vaginal approach has been chosen due to complexity and the need for exposure, then a Maylard incision is preferred. The Maylard incision should allow better exposure to the upper and midabdomen, along with improved access to the lateral pelvis. An emergent peripartum hysterectomy or one in which upper abdominal access is needed is best accomplished through a midline incision.

Several technical points about abdominal incisions, regardless of the type, apply. First, use of a skin marking pen may improve cosmetic results. A sketch of the proposed incision along with intermittent pen marking perpendicular to this incision may facilitate skin closure and lessen the chances of unequal skin edges. The scalpel should enter directly perpendicular to the skin and stay perpendicular through subsequent layers. Most surgeons feel that reoperation should be made through previous incisions. Parallel incisions often result in increased bleeding and may produce a devascularized wound. Minimal trauma to subcutaneous tissue, including overly aggressive hemostasis and "fat sweeping," provides a favorable environment for bacterial growth in devitalized tissue areas and will increase the incidence of fat necrosis, infection, and wound separation.

The obese patient presents a unique operative situation, beginning with incisional selection. Often the type of obesity dictates the choice of incision. A large hanging panniculus may allow a low transverse, noncrease-placed incision. Panniculectomy with or without abdominoplasty may also be indicated in these cases (71). Should a Pfannenstiel incision allow insufficient exposure, conversion to a Cherney incision may be preferable over the muscle-cutting Maylard technique. Theoretically, the vascular supply to the fascia is further sacrificed in the latter case.

When conversion to a Maylard incision is made, retraction of the rectus abdominus muscles occurs with poor muscle reapproximation at fascial closure (72). In the Maylard incision, ligation of the inferior epigastric vessels should be performed, which was not included in Maylard's initial description of the procedure (73). Others recommend subfascial closed drainage suction with Maylard incisions to minimize hematoma or seroma formation (74). A Maylard incision also allows lateral access into the peritoneum, which may often avoid midline subperitoneal adhesions from previous surgery. Usually, the peritoneum can be entered with the scalpel in a continuous motion.

Peritoneal elevation to visualize a diaphanous area in the peritoneum is unnecessary and no more successful in preventing inadvertent enterotomy or colotomy. After entrance into the peritoneal cavity, the upper abdomen is explored. Although laparoscopy offers visualization of this area, palpation of the kidneys, gall bladder, spleen, stomach, pancreas, appendix, and periaortic lymph nodes is forfeited. This speaks for another advantage of abdominal hysterectomy over a laparoscopic or vaginal approach.

Various self-retaining retractors can now be used for adequate exposure. Although the O'Sullivan-O'Connor or Balfour are most commonly used, the Bookwalter or Turner-Warwick ring self-retaining retractor allow blades of differing lengths and widths to be placed at any location in the wound (Figure 2-4). Application to the articulating arm can often be omitted due to its potential interference to surgeon mobility. With all retractors, cloth towels may be placed under the lateral blades to lessen compression of underlying pelvic sidewall structures that might result in possible femoral nerve compression. Lysis of adhesions will allow intestinal packing in a modest Trendelenburg position. Attempts to restore normal pelvic anatomy by lysis of adhesions will facilitate the performance of the hysterectomy. Attention is turned to the pelvis with palpation of the adnexae, cul de sac, and uterus. Thick-

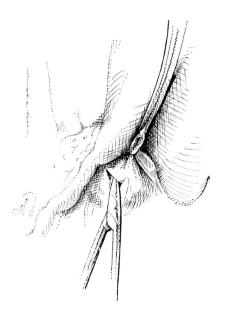

Figure 2-4 Creation of an opening in the broad ligament allows isolation of the ovarian vascular pedicle.

[17]

ness of remaining adhesions and mobility of the uterus are noted. Continuous traction-countertraction will facilitate exposure and lysis of adhesions, reduce blood loss, and expedite the procedure.

Technique

The first step in an abdominal hysterectomy is to isolate the round ligament by clamping it. Even with extensive disease or previous surgical distortion, the round ligament should be easily identifiable laterally. Occasionally, a previous uterine suspension will anatomically distort the location. In cases with distorted anatomy, a retroperitoneal dissection may begin at the level of the round ligaments. Identification, isolation, suture ligation, and incision of the uterine artery may be facilitated in this approach. Although during the retroperitoneal approach, pelvic vessels usually remain attached to the lateral pelvic sidewall, the ureter remains in the medial peritoneal reflection. In the routine approach, the round ligament is clamped, tied, and incised, allowing entrance into the retroperitoneal space at the broad ligament apex. The tied lateral stump of the broad ligament may be held for lateral retraction and eventual incorporation into the vaginal suspension. The anterior leaf of the broad ligament is incised and opened to the level of the bladder reflection from the lower uterine isthmus. Tension and traction on the peritoneal edges of the round ligament and uterus in opposite directions facilitate dissection within the loose areolar tissue. Bleeding is minimal if the correct plane of cleavage is found. Commonly the dissection is made more difficult when the incision is too high on the uterus.

The retroperitoneal space is now opened with transection of the above-discussed round ligament and then widened (Figure 2-4). Blunt dissection with the suction apparatus tip allows visualization of the iliac vessels and ureter. Retroperitoneal scarring from either endometriosis, previous pelvic surgery, or chronic pelvic infection may disallow blunt dissection. In these cases, sharp dissection beginning at the level of the pelvic brim over the common iliac vessels will allow exposure of the ureter as it falls medially in the leaf of peritoneum. A broad ligament myoma may also distort ureteral directions (Figure 2-5). Often, ureteral stinting will facilitate tactile sharp dissection in difficult cases. With the ureter visualized, mainly by peristalsis, or clearly palpable, either digital or instrumental pushing (right angle clamp) of the posterior leaf of the broad ligament in a forward manner will allow isolation of either the infundibulopelvic or utero-ovarian vessels.

Incision of this leaf of peritoneum is made, creating a window large enough to place three curved Kocher or similar clamps, incorporating either the uterine ovarian ligament and fallopian tube or, if the ovaries are to be removed, incorporating the infundibulopelvic ligament. The Kocher, Heaney, Heaney-Ballentine, and Masterson clamps are the most commonly used clamps for hysterectomy. Because of its width, head conformation, and ridge direction, the Masterson clamp is the least traumatic (Figure 2-6). Placement of three clamps may not be feasible in all cases without severe compromise to the vascular supply of

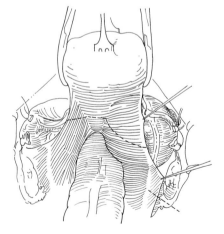

Figure 2-5 A broad ligament myoma may distort the normal ureteral course.

the mesovarium and mesosalpinx. In this case, passage of suture through the aperture in the broad liga ment with a tonsil hemostatic clamp may allow adequate pedicular ligation. Ideally, the placement of three clamps allows an incision to be made between the middle and most medial clamp (Figure 2-6). Then free suture ligation can be placed around the most lateral clamp and, upon its release, allow placement in the crushed ligamentous tissue. This manner of vessel ligation will avoid or decrease slippage and initial needle trauma of a vascular pedicle, as a transfixion suture ligature is then placed around both ends of the middle clamp. It should be noted that prior to tying the initial lateral suture ligature, the middle clamp should be minimally loosened to allow tight lateral ligation. Similar operative techniques should then occur on the contralateral side to limit subsequent blood loss during its dissection and increase uterine mobilization. The use of synthetic absorbable sutures, such as polyglactin (Vicryl) or polyglycolic acid (Dexon), offers several advantages over catgut sutures, including less tissue reactivity and greater resistance to breakage, thus allowing 2-0 or smaller ligatures for pelvic surgery. Trimming of vascular pedicles may reduce postoperative morbidity.

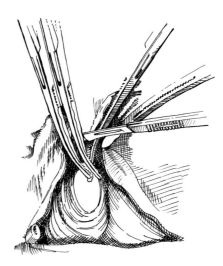

Figure 2-6 Triple clamp technique of the utero-ovarian vascular pedicle.

The next step involves separation of the bladder from the lower uterine segment. Use of blunt dissection and force may cause unnecessary trauma to the bladder, while distorting tissue planes and prohibiting clean access to the pubovesicocervical portion of the endopelvic fascia. The bladder must be taken down past the cervicovaginal junction. It should not be taken any further than necessary. Lateral to the base of the bladder and cervix is Santorini's vascular plexus. Dissection into this area should obviously be avoided due to profuse bleeding and ureteral proximity. Palpation of the cervix should lessen lateral dissection. Hypogastric ligation may be necessary to stop bleeding in this plexus. When extrafascial hysterectomy is necessary, further dissection is necessary to remove this fascia with the specimen.

NEXT PARA RESET

Sharp dissection of the posterior leaf of the broad ligament to the level of the uterosacral ligaments is now performed. Often dissection across the posterior cervix is delayed due to increased chances of bleeding. Instead, skeletonization of the uterine vessels is next performed. Exposure of the uterine vessels by sharp dissection is facilitated by contralateral uterine traction. Once the vessels are visualized, the triple clamp technique is again suggested (Figure 2-7). In an attempt to avoid ureteral injury, the lowest clamp is placed first and is bounced off the cervix at the level of the internal os until it may be placed at a right angle to the uterus. Palpation rather than visualization of the internal cervical os is suggested. The middle clamp is placed similarly. The most medial and third clamp prevents uterine back-bleeding and can be placed directly parallel to the longitudinal axis of the cervix. The vessels are cut with a scalpel between the medial and middle clamp. The incision is carried around the tip of the middle clamp. The uterine vessels are then double ligated, first around the lowest or lateral clamp, and then around the middle clamp. With laparoscopically assisted vaginal hysterectomy, perpendicular placement of either the electrocautery or stapling-cutting device is lessened by the nature of the endoscopic technique. The width of this device causes

Figure 2-7 Triple clamp technique of the uterine vessels at the level of the internal cervical os.

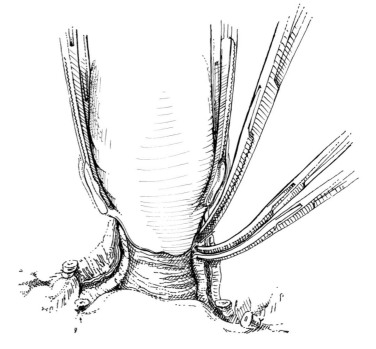

automatic stapling lateral to where clamp placement might be. As a result, the incidence of ureteral injury in these cases will most likely increase. If a hematoma results from unligated vessel slippage or vessel laceration into the broad ligament, control of bleeding should be immediate. Individual vessel location and clamping should be carried out. If unsuccessful, hypogastric artery ligation may be helpful.

Next, a straight hysterectomy clamp is placed medial to the previous uterine vesicular pedicle, downward and adjacent to the side of the uterus. Incision, leaving an ample wedge of upper cardinal ligament for suture ligation, is performed. Similar proceedings on the contralateral side are now performed. Uterine back-bleeding at the level of the uterine vessel should be minimized on the contralateral side. Once both right- and left-sided uterine vessles have been suture ligated, the peritoneum may be dissected off the cervix posteriorly with decreased amounts of bleeding. The uterosacral ligaments may now be clamped, cut, and suture ligated individually. Often, individual identification and suture ligation of these ligaments is difficult and omitted.

Attention is then turned anteriorly to the pubovesicocervical fascia. For the intrafascial hysterectomy technique, a V-shaped incision allows lateral retraction of the fascia from the cervix, which should be separated from the anterior surface of the cervix and bladder. This intrafascial technique lessens the incidence of vesicovaginal fistula formation (75). The remaining fascia also may be incorporated into support for the vagina, limiting the chances of eventual vaginal prolapse (76). The remaining dissection of the cardinal ligaments is accomplished by placement of straight clamps lateral to the cervix and beneath the pubovesicocervical fascia. Entrance into the vaginal fornix may occur during a progressive clamping, incising, and suture ligation of the cardinal ligament. Use of curved hysterectomy clamps will facilitate separation of uterus from vagina. Often, sharp entrance into the vagina may be accomplished by the scalpel. Separation of the cervix from the underly-

[20]

ing vagina is then performed. The entire removal of the cervix should be verified by inspection of the uterus prior to the handing-off of the specimen. Straight Kocher clamps can be used in the vaginal angles as the cervix is separated from the vagina for support and to limit retraction.

Once bleeding is controlled, the uterus should be bisected away from the operative field to rule out unsuspected endometrial disease, by which oophorectomy and nodal sampling may be indicated. A modification of the Richardson technique can be used to assist in vaginal suspension. The lateral angles of the vagina are transfixed to their respective cardinal ligament pedicles. Often, the vaginal angle bleeds, and its incorporation into this transfixion lessens this possibility (Figure 2-8). The exposed upper margin of the vagina is run with continuous locking suture. The vaginal cuff is left open to allow drainage of serosanguinous fluid (77). Extraperitonealization of vascular pedicles will allow easy and early recognition of their bleeding through the vagina should bleeding occur. Since a closed vaginal cuff allows midline accumulation of large quantities of serosanguinous fluid, the cuff is routinely left open. However, reapproximation of the vaginal cuff by closure may lessen vaginal apex granulation tissue formation by limiting closure by secondary intention without increasing postoperative morbidity (78). Others who leave the vaginal cuff open pay particular attention to suture placement, running the cuff in a Lembert manner, avoiding the vaginal mucosa so that no suture actually appears in the vagina. The use of the T-tube transvaginal cuff drainage fails to equal the success of prophylactic antibiotic use in reducing febrile morbidity (79). In addition, there is no additive effect of T-tube cuff drainage with prophylactic antibiotic use (80).

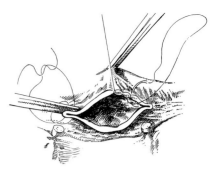

Figure 2-8 Transfixation and incorporation of the lateral vaginal angles.

Support to the vaginal vault may be intensified by more than lateral margin transfixion to the cardinal ligament and perivaginal fascia. A McCall posterior culdoplasty, which involves incorporation and transfixion of both uterosacral ligaments to the posterior vaginal fornix, may be performed. Further suspension of the vagina is afforded by including anterior vagina, cardinal ligament, round ligament, uterosacral ligament, and posterior vagina. Incorporation of the uterine ovarian ligaments in this suspension would most likely lead to medial, supravaginal displacement of the ovaries, with the increased risk of dyspareunia. Fallopian tube prolapse is much more common after vaginal hysterectomy, but closure of the peritoneum over the bladder may help prevent herniation of these structures, and reperitonealization is most likely unnecessary (81). Reperitonealization, in addition to increasing operative time, may also increase the possibility of ureteral kinking by incorporation of the peritoneum and may also allow inadvertent needle passage distal to a previously ligated vascular pedicle. Peritoneal defects will be closed by natural reperitonealization within two to three days (82). A Moschowitz culdoplasty may be used to reduce a deep posterior cul-de-sac potential future enterocele formation. In the culdoplasty, a purse string nonpermanent suture begins at the nadir of the posterior cul-de-sac and is worked upward, incorporating the uterosacral ligaments, posterior vagina, lateral peritoneum, and sigmoid colon serosa

(83). Prior to closure, water can be placed into the pelvis and individual bleeders can be visualized clearly through the water. In this way, water allows localization of bleeders as well as a bacterial diluent prior to closure. Closure is then performed in the standard method. Peritoneal closure may be indicated in a Maylard incision by preventing serosanguinous fluid seepage from the cut rectus muscle into the pelvic cavity, but in other incisions, it is probably unnecessary (84). Prior to termination of the operation, often during fascial closure, an ampule of indigo carmine may be given intravenously. The Foley catheter is now removed from the bladder. With the patient in Allen stirrups, easy access to the urethra is allowed. Simple cystoscopy with either sorbitol or glycine bladder irrigation is then set up. Using a 30°-angle cystoscope, visualization of the ureteral orifices, posteriorly and proximal to the urethral sphincter, is performed. The release of indigo carmine from each orifice confirms ureteral patency. While this procedure is probably not necessary in all hysterectomies, it allows the gynecologist familiarity with the cystoscope, and its similarities to hysteroscopic use become quite apparent. Cystoscopy also allows one to note bladder mucosal anatomy for comparison to future possible pathological cases, e.g., cervical or endometrial carcinoma.

The difficult hysterectomy

Two scenarios often present especially technically difficult abdominal hysterectomies: the emergent peripartum hysterectomy and the abdominal hysterectomy involving severe posterior cul-de-sac adhesions with obliteration of the space due to either endometriosis or pelvic inflammatory disease. The peripartum hysterectomy presents two main problems: the ability to decrease rapid hemorrhage and the difficulty in delineating the cervix from the vagina. In the case of cul-de-sac adhesions, a "backwards" hysterectomy is often performed, excising the uterus off the rectum to lessen the chances of inadvertent rectosigmoid entrance.

Emergent cesarean hysterectomy

After delivery of the infant and placenta, closure of the uterine incision is completed. This reduced total blood loss and attempts to ensure a dry operative field for the rest of the procedure. Next, the operative procedure is performed similarly to in the nonpregnant state. Obviously, pelvic vascular engorgement allows the opportunity for easy hemorrhage. For example, Sampson's artery, paralleling the round ligament, must be included in the suture ligation or profuse bleeding will occur. Additionally, stretching of the broad ligaments during pregnancy and their nontaut state postpartum potentiate lateral clamp placement with endangerment to the ureters. Placement of the entire length of the clamp adjacent to the uterus lessens the potential for ureteral injury (85). Clamping of the uterine vessels proceeds after adequate skeletonization has been performed. Sharp rather than blunt dissection of the

[22]

bladder is crucial. Blunt dissection will often result in hemorrhage due to pericervical vein rupture.

One of the most difficult parts of the cesarean hysterectomy is identification of the vaginal cervical border. This delineation is difficult after advanced labor with maximal or near maximal cervical dilation. Several techniques facilitate this separation. Often, a large ring forceps clamp can be placed transvaginally on the cervical lip at the start of the hysterectomy and released after entrance into the vagina has been accomplished. Another technique involves performing an initial supracervical hysterectomy. The surgeon's fingers are then placed within the vagina and, moving the hand cephalad, the cervical lip may be palpated. Bleeding often occurs from the vascular vagina.

"Backwards" hysterectomy

As discussed, severe rectovaginal or sigmoid uterine adhesions prevent perceived performance of the hysterectomy in the usual manner. In these cases, the hysterectomy might be best performed from the cervix toward the uterine fundus. In this approach, isolation of the uterine arteries is mandatory. Opening the peritoneum lateral to the common iliac artery allows the ureter to fall medially within the peritoneal reflection. The bifurcation of the common iliac artery is identified into the internal (hypogastric) and external iliac vessels around the sacroiliac joint, and dissection is carried downward along the hypogastric artery. The hypogastric artery supplies flow to the viscera of the pelvis. Approximately three to four centimeters after separating from the external iliac, the hypogastric divides into an anterior and posterior division. Injury to the posterior division, which supplies the lateral sacral, iliolumbar, and superior gluteal arteries, should be avoided. The anterior division of the hypogastric artery is then followed forward until the uterine artery is identified. The uterine artery can be identified as it courses over the ureter. To facilitate this identification, ureteral dissection must be accomplished. A right-angle clamp placed over the ureter will allow its separation from surrounding tissue. Once the uterine artery traverses over the ureter, it may be ligated at this point.

Next, attention is turned to the anterior cervix. The bladder peritoneal reflection is dissected from and mobilized off the cervix in the usual manner. Intrafascial dissection again will lessen the possibility of bladder trauma. At this time, the scalpel is used to sharply enter the anterior vagina, and the anterior cervix is dissected from the vagina. Once the entire cervical os is within view, the anatomical dissection is toward the fundus. Areas of uterine serosa may be left on the large bowel, but colotomy is prevented. Bleeding is minimized due to the previous uterine artery ligation.

Conclusions

Newer medicinal and surgical conservative therapies have lessened the necessity to perform abdominal hysterectomy. Only certain conditions

[23]

dictate an abdominal approach, occasionally emergently. As resident teaching and attention is geared more toward laparoscopic surgery and away from laparotomy, the skills necessary to perform an abdominal hysterectomy may deteriorate. Many modifications in the technique have been made since the first successful abdominal hysterectomy in 1850 (86). Changes were most often the result of well-designed comparative studies. The question remains as to whether newer endoscopic modalities will also undergo such rigorous examination and survive under similar scrutiny.

References

1 Pokras R, Hufnagel VG. Hysterectomy in the United States, 1965–84. AJPN 1988;78:852–853.

2 McCoy NL, Davidson JM. A longitudinal study of the effects of menopause on sexuality. Maturitas 1985;7:203–206.

3 Kjerulff K, Langenberg P, Guzinski G. The socioeconomic correlates of hysterectomies in the United States. Am J Public Health 1993;83:106–108.

4 McCarthy EG, Kamons AS. Voluntary and mandatory presurgical screening programs: an analysis of their implications. Presented at the American Federation for Clinical Research, Clinical Epidemiology, Health Care Research, Atlantic City, New Jersey, May 2, 1972.

5 Finkel ML, Finkel DJ. The effect of a second opinion program on hysterectomy performance. Med Care 1990;28:776–783.

6 Reiter RC, Gambone JC, Lench JB. Appropriateness of hysterectomies performed for multiple preoperative indications. Obstet Gynecol 1992;80:902–905.

7 Gambone JC, Reiter RC, Lench JB, Moore JG. The impact of a quality assurance process on the frequency and confirmation rate of hysterectomy. Am J Obstet Gynecol 1990;163:545–550.

8 Thompson JD, Birch HW. Indications for hysterectomy. Clin Obstet Gynecol 1981;24:1245–1258.

9 Hysterectomies in the United States, 1965–84. Vital Health Stat 1988;13.

10 Cramer SF, Patel D. The frequency of uterine leiomyomas. Am J Clin Path 1990;94:435–438.

11 Wintherspoon JR, Butler VW. The etiology of uterine fibroids with special reference to the frequency of their occurrence on the negro: a hypothesis. Surg Gynecol Obstet 1934;58:57–61.

12 Cramer DW, Wilson E, Stillman RJ, et al. The relation of endometriosis to menstrual characteristics, smoking, and exercise. JAMA 1986;255:1904–1908.

13 Quality assurance in obstetrics and gynecology. Washington, D.C.: American College of Obstetricians and Gynecologists 1989;28.

14 Friedman AJ, Haas ST. Should uterine size be indication for surgical intervention in women with myomas? Am J Obstet Gynecol 1993;168:751–755.

15 Giudice LC, Jacobs A, Pineda J, Bell CE, Lippmann L. Serum levels of CA-125 in patients with endometriosis. Fertil Steril 1986;45:876–891.

16 Dudiak CM, Turner DA, Patel SK, Archie JT, Silver B, Norusis M. Uterine leiomyomas in the infertile patient: preoperative localization with MR imaging versus US and hysterosalpingography. Radiology 1988;167:627–630.

17 Reiter RC, Wagner PL, Gambone JC. Routine hysterectomy for large asymptomatic uterine leiomyomata: a reappraisal. Obstet Gynecol 1992;79:481–484.

18 Schloff WD, Zerhoune EA, Hutch JA, Chen J, Danewood MD, Rock JA. A placebo-controlled trial of a depot gonadotropin-releasing hormone analogue (Leuprolide) in the treatment of uterine leiomyomata. Obstet Gynecol 1989;74:856–862.

19 Matta W, Stahite I, Shaw RW, Campbell S. Doppler assessment of uterine blood flow changes in patients with fibroid receiving the gonadotropin-releasing hormone agonist buserelin. Fertil Steril 1988;49:1083–1085.

20 Lumsden MA, West CP, Baird DT. Goserelin therapy before surgery for uterine fibroids. Lancet 1987;1:36–37.

21 Stovall TG, Ling FW, Henry LC, Woodruff MR. A randomized trial evaluating

leuprolide acetate before hysterectomy as treatment for leiomyomas. Am J Obstet Gynecol 1991;164:1420–1425.

22 Friedman AJ. Treatment of leiomyomata uteri with short-term leuprolide followed by leuprolide plus estrogen-progestin hormone replacement therapy for two years: a pilot study. Fertil Steril 1989;51:526–528.

23 Coutinho EM, Concalves MT. Long-term treatment of leiomyomas with gestrinone. Fertil Steril 1989;51:939–946.

24 Coutinho EM. Gestrinone in the treatment of myomas. Acta Obstet Gynecol Scand Suppl 1989;150:39–46.

25 Meyer WR, Mayer AR, Diamond MP, Carcangiu ML, Schwartz PE, DeCherney AH. Unsuspected leiomyosarcoma: treatment with a gonadotropin-releasing hormone analogue. Obstet Gynecol 1990;75:529–531.

26 Loong EPL, Wong FWS. Uterine leiomyosarcoma diagnosed during treatment with agonist of luteinizing hormone releasing hormone for presumed uterine fibroid. Fertil Steril 1990;54:530–534.

27 Meyerovitz MF, Lobel SM, Harrington DP, Bengston JM. Preoperative uterine artery embolization in cervical pregnancy." JUIR 1991;2:95–97.

28 Farabow WS, Fulton JW, Fletcher V, et al. Cervical pregnancy treated with methotrarate. NC Med J 1983;44:91–93.

29 Yankowitz J, Leake J, Huggins G, Gazaway P, Gates E. Cervical ectopic pregnancy: review of the literature and report of a case treated by single-dose methotrexate therapy. Obstet Gynecol Surv 1988;45:405–413.

30 Oyer R, Tarakjian ID, Lef-Toaff A, et al. Treatment of cervical pregnancy with methotrexate. Obstet Gynecol 1988;71:469–471.

31 Wheeler JH, Malinak LR. Recurrent endometriosis: incidence, management, and prognosis. Am J Obstet Gynecol 1983;146:247–251.

32 Andrews WC, Larson GD. Endometriosis treatment with hormonal pseudopregnancy and/or reoperation. Am J Obstet Gynecol 1974;118:643–649.

33 Andrews WC. Medical versus surgical treatment of endometriosis. Clin Obstet Gynecol 1980;23:917–924.

34 Sampson JA. Heterotopic or misplaced endometrial tissue. Am J Obstet Gynecol 1925;10:649–656.

35 Cashman BZ. Hysterectomy with preservation of ovarian tissue in the treatment of endometriosis. Am J Obstet Gynecol 1945;49:484–493.

36 Williams TJ, Pratt JH. Endometriosis in 1,000 consecutive celiotomies: incidence and management. Am J Obstet Gynecol 1977;129:245–250.

37 Sheets JL, Symmonds RE, Banner EA. Conservative surgical management of endometriosis. Obstet Gynecol 1964;23:625–631.

38 Williams TJ. The role of surgery in the management of endometriosis. Mayo Clin Proc 1975;50:198–203.

39 Kaminski PF, Sorosky JI, Mandell MJ, Broadstreet RP, Zanio PJ. Clomiphene citrate stimulation as an adjunct in locating ovarian tissue in ovarian remnant syndrome. Obstet Gynecol 1990;76:924–926.

40 Ovarian remnant syndrome: difficulties in diagnosis and management. Obstet Gynecol Surv 1990;45:151–156.

41 Scott RB, Telinde RW. External endometriosis—the scourge of the private patient. Ann Surg 1950;131:697–720.

42 Scott RB, Burt JH. Clinical external endometriosis: fifteen years experience at University Hospitals of Cleveland. So Med J 1962;55:129–136.

43. Ranney B. Endometriosis III. Complete operations. Am J Obstet Gynecol 1971;109:1137–1145.

44 Chestnut DH, Eden RD, Stanley SA, Parker RT. Peripartum hysterectomy: a review of cesarean and postpartum hysterectomy. Obstet Gynecol 1985;65:365–370.

45 Yancey MK, Harlass FE, Benson W, Brady K. The perioperative morbidity of scheduled cesarean hysterectomy. Obstet Gynecol 1993;81:206–210.

46 Stanco LM, Schrimmer BB, Paul HP, Mistell DR. Emergency peripartum hysterectomy and associated risk factors. Am J Obstet Gynecol 1993;168:879–883.

47 Diciler RC, Greenspan JR, Strauss LT, et al. Complications of abdominal and vaginal hysterectomy among women of reproductive age in the United States. Am J Obstet Gynecol 1982;144:841–847.

48 Lee NC, Dicker RC, Rubin GL, Ory HW. Confirmation of the preoperative diagnosis for hysterectomy. Am J Obstet Gynecol 1984;150:283–287.

49 Melzack R. Neurophysiological foundations of pain. In: Stornbach RA, ed. The psychology of pain, 2nd ed. New York: Raven Press, 1986;1:24.

50 Renaer M, Vertommen H, Hijs P. Psychological aspects of chronic pelvic pain in women. Am J Obstet Gynecol 1979;134:75–80.

51 Magni G, Salmy A, Delio D, Ceola A. Chronic pelvic pain and depression. Psychopathology 1984;17:132–136.

52 Gambone JC, Reiter RC. Nonsurgical management of chronic pelvic pain: a multidisciplinary approach. Clin Obstet Gynecol 1990;33:205–211.

53 Mitchell DG. Benign diseases of the uterus and ovaries. Applications of magnetic resonance imaging. Rad Clin N Amer 1992;30:777–787.

54 Stovall TG, Ling FW, Crawford DA. Hysterectomy for chronic pelvic pain of presumed uterine etiology. Obstet Gynecol 1990;75:676–679.

55 Groodnagh LT, Shuck JM. Risks, options, and informed consent for blood transfusion in elective surgery. Am J Surg 1990;159:602–609.

56 Richards C, Kolins J, Trindale. (1) Antologus transfusion—transmitted *Yersinia enterocolitica*." JAMA 1992;268:152–154.

57 HERS Newsletter. Hysterectomy educational resources and services. 1985;2:1–6.

58 Oldenhave A, Jaszmann LJB, Evergerd WT, Haspels AA. Hysterectomized women with ovarian conservation report more severe climacteric complaints than do normal climacteric women of similar age. Am J Obstet Gynecol 1993;168:765–771.

59 Siddle N, Sarrel P, Whitehead M. The effect of hysterectomy on the age at ovarian failure: identification of a subgroup of women with premature loss of ovarian function and literature review. Fertil Steril 1987;47:94–100.

60 Martin RL, Roberts WV, Clayton PS. Psychiatric status after hysterectomy. A one-year prospective follow-up. JAMA 1980;244:350–353.

61 Hayek LF, Emerson JM, Gardner AMN. A placebo-controlled trial of the effect of two preoperative baths or showers with corhexidine detergent on postoperative wound infection rates. J Hosp Infec 1987;10:165–173.

62 Aristey MS, Jones AP. Preparation of the vagina for surgery. JAMA 1981;245:839–841.

63 Zakut H, Lotan M, Bracha Y. Vaginal preparation with povidone-iodine before abdominal hysterectomy: a comparison with antibiotic prophylaxis. Clin Exp Obstet Gynecol 1987;14:1–5.

64 Bird BJ, Chrisp DB, Jerimgeour G. Extensive preoperative shaving: a costly exercise. NZ Med J 1984;97:727–730.

65 Seropian R, Reynolds BM. Wound infections after preoperative depilatory versus razor preparation. Am J Surg 1971;122:251–256.

66 Duff P. Antibiotic prophylaxis for abdominal hysterectomy. Obstet Gynecol 1980;60:25–29.

67 Shapiro M, Munoz A, Tuger I, Thoenbaum S, Polk FB. Risk factors for infection at the operative site after abdominal or vaginal hysterectomy. N Engl J Med 1991;307:1661–1666.

68 Houang ET. Antibiotic prophylaxis in hysterectomy and induced abortion. Drugs 1991;41:19–37.

69 Thompson JD. Hysterectomy. In: Thompson JD, Rock JA, eds. Telinde's operative gynecology. 7th ed. Philadelphia: JB Lippincott Co. 1992;663–738.

70 Capen CV. Gynecologic surgery: preoperative evaluation. Clin Obstet Gynecol 1988;31:673–685.

71 Masterson BJ. Selection of incisions for gynecologic procedures. Surg Clin N Amer 1991;71:1041–1051.

72 Thompson JD. Incisions for gynecologic surgery. In: Thompson JD, Rock JA, eds. Telinde's operative gynecology. 7th ed. Philadelphia: Lippincott Co. 1992;239–277.

73 Maylard AE. Direction of abdominal incisions. Br Med J 1907;2:895–901.

74 Helmkamp BF, Krebs HB. The Maylard incision in gynecologic surgery. Am J Obstet Gynecol 1990;163:1554–1557.

75 Falk HC. Prevention of vesicovaginal fistula in total hysterectomy for benign disease. Obstet Gynecol 1967;29:865–868.

76 Jaszczak, Evans TN. Intrafascial abdominal and vaginal hysterectomy: a reappraisal. Obstet Gynecol 1982;59:435–444.

77 Gray LA. Techniques of abdominal total hysterectomy, with report of three methods used in 1,000 cases. Am J Obstet Gynecol 1958;75:334–347.

78 Johnson JR, Gardner WN, Diddle AW. Management of the vaginal cuff. Am J Obstet Gynecol 1963;87:951–955.

79 Wijma J, Kavaer FM, Van Saere MKF, varde Wiel HBM, Jansens J. Antibiotics and suction drainage as prophylaxis in vaginal and abdominal hysterectomy. Obstet Gynecol 1987;70:384–388.

80 Poulsen HK, Bonl J. T-tube suction drainage and/or prophylactic two-dose metronidazole in abdominal hysterectomy. Obstet Gynecol 1984;63:291–294.

81 Sumathy V, Baucum K. Prolapse of the fallopian tube following abdominal hysterectomy. Int J Gynecol Obstet 1975;13:273–276.

82 Raftery AT. Regeneration of parietal and visceral peritoneum. Brit J Surg 1973;60: 293–299.

83 Moschcowitz AV. The pathogensis, anatomy, and cure of prolapse of the rectum. Surg Gynecol Obstet 1912;15:7–21.

84 Pietrantori M, Parsons MT, O'Brien WF. Peritoneal closure or nonclosure at cesarean section. Obstet Gynecol 1991;77:293–296.

85 Iffy L, Apuzzio JJ, Vintzeleos AM. Operative obstetrics. New York: McGraw-Hill, Inc. 1992;415–418.

86 Benrubi GI. History of hysterectomy. J Fla Med Assoc 1988;75:533.

3 Hysterectomy: Vaginal Approach

DEIRDRE ROBINSON & THOMAS G. STOVALL

Hysterectomy is the second most commonly performed operation in the United States each year despite increasing opportunities for nonsurgical and minimally invasive management of many gynecologic diseases. As a result, gynecologists must remain abreast of surgical advances as well as the risks and benefits of both the abdominal and vaginal approaches to hysterectomy. The vast majority of the 650,000 annual hysterectomies are performed abdominally, with only 28% of all hysterectomies performed via the vaginal route (1). Proponents of vaginal surgery argue that vaginal hysterectomy invokes less morbidity, decreases hospitalization and recovery time, and reduces medical costs when compared with abdominal hysterectomy. With careful preoperative selection, up to one half of all hysterectomies could be completed vaginally (2). This concept is echoed in the adage that "the only indications for an abdominal hysterectomy are the contraindications to vaginal hysterectomy" (3). This chapter will review the advantages of vaginal hysterectomy, standard surgical approaches, and recent advances in surgical management.

Safety of vaginal hysterectomy

Historically, the vaginal approach to hysterectomy was considered inferior to abdominal hysterectomy. The concept of operating "in the dark" and an associated increased morbidity with vaginal hysterectomy made abdominal hysterectomy the procedure of choice. Until relatively recently, few studies were available to compare the risks and benefits of vaginal and abdominal hysterectomy.

In 1951, Leventhal compared a series of 300 vaginal hysterectomies to 300 abdominal hysterectomies to evaluate the morbidity of each procedure (4). The surgical route was chosen by the operator based on clinical judgment and surgical skill. Experienced surgeons performed vaginal hysterectomy 50% of the time while more junior surgeons utilized the vaginal route 25% of the time. Oophorectomy accompanied hysterectomy in 7.3% of vaginal cases and 82.3% of abdominal hysterectomy cases. Morbidity was primarily attributed to urinary retention, urinary tract infection, and unexplained fevers. Of interest, both episodes of ureteral injury occurred during an abdominal hysterectomy. The morbidity rate for vaginal hysterectomy ranged from 38.1% for simple hysterectomy to 52.5% for vaginal hysterectomy with removal of

the adnexa and/or colporrhaphy. The morbidity rate for vaginal procedures was significantly higher than the morbidity rate of 27.3% for all
abdominal procedures. The authors concluded that despite increased
morbidity, vaginal hysterectomy did have a role in gynecologic surgery,
albeit a limited one.

Enthusiasm for vaginal hysterectomy remained tempered in 1971,
when White reviewed his series of 300 abdominal and 300 vaginal hysterectomies (5). While overall morbidity rates were similar for both
groups, the etiology of postoperative complications was different for the
vaginal and abdominal routes of hysterectomy. Febrile morbidity occurred in 55% of vaginal hysterectomies as compared with 36% of abdominal procedures. Conversely, abdominal hysterectomy was more
often associated with wound infections, ileus, and blood transfusions.
As no distinct advantage in morbidity was present over either route of
hysterectomy, neither procedure could be recommended over the other.
Thus, the route of hysterectomy was left to the surgeon, taking into
account clinical judgment and level of surgical skill.

A study comparing the surgical indications for and outcome of vaginal and abdominal hysterectomy was finally performed by Dicker et al.
in 1982 (6). The Collaborative Review of Sterilization project prospectively evaluated 1,851 reproductive age women undergoing vaginal or
abdominal hysterectomy in a multicenter observational trial. The route
of hysterectomy was chosen by the attending surgeon, with the most
common indications for hysterectomy being fibroids, genital prolapse,
and endometriosis. Abdominal hysterectomy was chosen in 72% of
cases, and vaginal hysterectomy was used in 28%. The route of approach was changed intraoperatively from vaginal to abdominal in 1%
of vaginal hysterectomies when it was technically not feasible to use the
vaginal route. Overall, morbidity was 1.7 times greater with abdominal
hysterectomy than vaginal hysterectomy. Although the vaginal route
had lower morbidity, an unplanned major surgical procedure was more
often required. Additional surgery was performed in 2.5% of vaginal
cases and 1% of abdominal cases. All of the ureteral injuries occurred in
the abdominal group. To determine if selection bias had influenced
morbidity with either procedure, 264 cases were reviewed. All were
deemed appropriate for either vaginal or abdominal hysterectomy based
on preoperative information. The morbidity of 150 women who underwent abdominal hysterectomy was compared with 114 women who underwent vaginal hysterectomy. The complication rates of these sub-
groups were not different from the respective groups as a whole. The
relative risk of morbidity for abdominal hysterectomy as compared with
vaginal hysterectomy was 2:1 in the group of patients in whom either
route would have been appropriate. Vaginal hysterectomy overall was
now demonstrated to be less morbid than the standard of abdominal
hysterectomy. The authors surmised that the overall morbidity with
vaginal hysterectomy could be reduced by the routine use of prophylactic antibiotics and, thus, an associated decline in febrile morbidity.

In addition to decreased morbidity, this study also demonstrated that
vaginal hysterectomy results in less patient discomfort, earlier hospital

discharge, and faster recovery than abdominal hysterectomy. Thus, vaginal hysterectomy should be the procedure of choice unless an indication for abdominal hysterectomy exists.

The common indications for choosing the abdominal route for hysterectomy include (1) lack of uterine mobility, (2) uterine size greater than the equivalent of 12 weeks gestation, (3) presence of an adnexal tumor in which malignancy is a distinct possibility, (4) a massively contracted bony pelvis, (5) a clear-cut need for exploring the remainder of the abdomen, or (6) lack of surgeon experience and enthusiasm for the vaginal approach (3).

Preoperative use of gonadotropin-releasing hormone agonists

Leiomyomata uteri is the most common indication for hysterectomy, and inherent to most leiomyomata that require surgical management is an increase in uterine size (6). The practical solution is most often abdominal hysterectomy. A method to preoperatively reduce uterine size would offer greater opportunity to perform a vaginal rather than an abdominal hysterectomy.

Leiomyomata are known to be hormone-dependent tumors that can be reduced in size with administration of gonadotropin-releasing hormone (GnRH) agonists. Stovall et al. conducted a randomized trial to determine if preoperative GnRH agonist treatment of fibroid uteri could allow a vaginal hysterectomy instead of an abdominal approach (7). Fifty women with uteri clinically judged to be 14–18 weeks' size were randomized to 25 control patients and 25 patients to receive pretreatment with GnRH agonist. Treated patients received either 3.75 mg IM Lupron monthly or 0.5 mg/day subcutaneous Lupron daily for two months. Control patients proceeded directly to hysterectomy. Uterine size was evaluated pre- and post-treatment by clinical exam and ultrasound. Following GnRH agonist therapy, mean uterine size decreased from 15.7 to 11.4 weeks, and 76% of treated patients were considered to be candidates for vaginal hysterectomy. The uterus was successfully removed vaginally in 68% of these patients. Both the control and GnRH agonist groups had similar operative times and blood loss. Mean duration of hospitalization and convalescence was significantly shorter in the GnRH agonist-treated group. Pretreatment of leiomyomata uteri with GnRH agonist significantly reduces uterine size and allows an increased utilization of vaginal hysterectomy in those patients with a pretreatment uterine size of 14–18 weeks' gestational size.

Laparoscopically assisted vaginal hysterectomy

The ability to perform a vaginal hysterectomy can be limited by uterine size, pelvic adhesions, endometriosis, and reduced uterine mobility. An alternative to the difficult vaginal hysterectomy or conventional abdominal approach lies with the laparoscopically assisted vaginal hysterectomy (LAVH). Laparoscopy has been used in varying degrees, from simple assessment of the condition of the pelvis to lysis of pelvic adhesions to total laparoscopic hysterectomy. The laparoscope is most commonly used to facilitate a difficult vaginal hysterectomy by laparoscopic ligation of the infundibulopelvic ligaments and uterine vessels. The resultant increase in uterine mobility and ligation of the ovarian pedicles may allow vaginal removal of the uterus, which otherwise might have required an abdominal procedure.

While experience with advanced laparoscopic surgery is steadily increasing, little data is available as to the appropriate and effective use of these skills. Laparoscopically assisted vaginal hysterectomy was recently compared with standard vaginal hysterectomy in a randomized trial (8). Twenty-eight of 56 candidates scheduled for vaginal hysterectomy were randomized to undergo LAVH. The operative laparoscope was used to ligate the infundibulopelvic and cardinal ligaments and uterine vessels, with the remainder of the hysterectomy completed vaginally. The patients undergoing LAVH had longer operating time, increased requirements for pain medication, and a 60% increase in operating costs. LAVH offered no advantage over standard vaginal hysterectomy in patients who could otherwise undergo vaginal hysterectomy. Therefore, LAVH should not take the place of vaginal hysterectomy. Further study is needed to determine the role of LAVH in patients who would otherwise require abdominal surgery.

Outpatient vaginal hysterectomy

If the vaginal route has been selected for hysterectomy, consideration should be given to the possibility of an outpatient procedure. The healthy patient who has undergone a vaginal hysterectomy can now have the option of ambulatory surgery. The advantages of decreased hospitalization costs and the ability to remain close to family and recover in familiar surroundings are appealing to many women. This issue must be addressed preoperatively to allow adequate preparation and education of the patient and family for an early discharge. A prospective trial evaluating the feasibility and safety of outpatient vaginal hysterectomy was conducted by Stovall et al. in 1992 (9). Thirty-five healthy, motivated women with good home support were entered into the trial. Home health care support was provided by means of nursing visits and physician telephone contact. Nursing assessment included general evaluation, vital signs, and blood counts. The majority of the patients were satisfied with their outpatient hysterectomy and were happy with the early discharge arrangements. Two women required rehospitalization, one for treatment of a spinal headache and another for a cuff cellulitis. Four patients were dissatisfied with the level of pain control at home, and the two patients requiring readmission were unhappy with the same-day discharge arrangements in general. Outpatient vaginal hysterectomy can be a positive experience for many women if conducted in the setting of careful patient selection and adequate medical and family support.

Vasoconstrictive agents

The risks of intraoperative blood loss are ever increasing both for the patient and the surgeon. The current concern over blood-borne infectious agents has greatly increased the risks of blood transfusion and intraoperative contamination. Any mechanism to help avoid blood loss, transfusion, and surgical exposure is welcome for many gynecologic surgeons. One of the initial steps during vaginal hysterectomy is incision of the cervix portio, which often results in persistent bleeding from exposed submucosa and peritoneal vessels. In an effort to secure hemostasis, the cervical mucosa is often injected with a dilute solution of epinephrine. In the 1950s, Lazar presented a report of the use of dilute (1:1000) epinephrine infiltration during a variety of vaginal procedures (10). The decision to use infiltration and the volume of epinephrine injected was left to the operator. Intraoperative estimated blood loss was compared between the injected and noninjected patients. The mean estimated blood loss during vaginal hysterectomy of patients without infiltration was 305 cc and with infiltration was 755 cc. Similar results of decreased blood loss with infiltration were described for anterior and posterior colporrhaphy as well as Manchester operations. No information was available as to the indications for use of epinephrine by a particular surgeon or if infiltration was more likely to be used in more difficult cases. No significant morbidity was reported, leading to the conclusion that infiltration with dilute epinephrine was a safe and effective procedure.

A randomized trial of saline versus dilute epinephrine injection during vaginal hysterectomy was conducted by England et al. in 1983 (11). Two hundred women were randomized either to injection with normal saline or a solution of 1:200,000 epinephrine into the mucosa and submucosal tissue of the cervix. Outcome measures included intraoperative blood loss and postoperative vaginal cuff infection. The mean estimated blood loss of the control group of 310 ml was not significantly different than the mean loss of 280 ml in the epinephrine-treated group. No significant difference was present in the incidence of blood transfusion or in the change in hematocrit of the two groups. Vaginal cuff infections occurred in 11% of patients treated with epinephrine and only 2% of control patients, giving a relative risk of developing a cuff infection of 5.5 ($p < 0.1$) if epinephrine was used. This randomized trial of injection of epinephrine during vaginal hysterectomy reveals no improvement in blood loss and a markedly increased risk of vaginal cuff infection. Based on this data, infiltration with epinephrine cannot be encouraged and other alternatives for cuff hemostasis, such as hemostatic sutures, should be considered.

Ureteral identification

Injury to the ureter can occur during both abdominal and vaginal hysterectomy with an incidence of 0.25 to 3.0% (12). The actual rate of injury is difficult to determine as many ureteral injuries are unrecognized or unreported. In general, ureteral injury does occur 1.5 times more frequently during an abdominal hysterectomy than during vaginal hysterectomy. Initial studies to identify the ureter during vaginal hysterectomy were conducted by Hofmeister in 1961 (13). Using intravenous pyelogram, x-ray, and cinefluorography, the ureter was visualized with each clamp placement during the operation. The authors found that ureteral dissection was difficult and that the ureter was difficult to identify or palpate, even after placement of ureteral stents. Radiographic studies confirmed that the ureter remained in close proximity to the operating field for much of the hysterectomy. The ureter was less than 1 cm away from the infundibulopelvic ligament clamp during removal of the tube and ovary and was at greatest risk during an anterior colporrhaphy. The distance between the ureters and the surgical field could be best maximized by placing continuous anterior retraction on the bladder and downward traction on the cervix during the initial stages of the vaginal hysterectomy. This maneuver allowed the ureters to be pulled up and away from the uterosacral and cardinal ligaments. This careful documentation of the course of the ureter provided valuable insight into the risk of ureteral injury during vaginal surgery.

Cruikshank described a technique of vaginal dissection and ureteral identification allowing for direct visualization and palpation of the ureter during vaginal hysterectomy (12). Forty consecutive patients underwent vaginal hysterectomy for benign disease and had concurrent dissection and identification of the ureters. Following entry into both the anterior and posterior cul-de-sac, the bladder was elevated and retracted anteriorly. The infundibulopelvic ligament and the hypogastric artery were then identified by palpation and the ureters located between these vessels. Retroperitoneal dissection under the base of the bladder was then performed to identify the distal portion of the ureters. This was accomplished by placing traction on the bladder pillars and undermining the peritoneum 4–5 cm to allow visualization and palpation of the distal ureters and the ureterovesical junction. The hysterectomy was then completed in a standard fashion. The ureters were successfully identified bilaterally in all but three patients, two of whom were obese. Complications were limited to an episode of cuff cellulitis, one patient with persistent cuff bleeding, and a bladder laceration during anterior colporrhaphy. Identification of the ureters during vaginal hysterectomy is technically feasible and appears to be associated with low morbidity. It is an invaluable skill that should be learned by all gynecologic surgeons.

Operative techniques

The standard Heaney technique is the most common method taught and utilized for vaginal hysterectomy (14). This approach involves direct entry into the peritoneal cavity with subsequent sequential ligation of the ligaments and vascular pedicles in reverse order of the standard abdominal hysterectomy. Many variations on this original method have been described to modify this technique and adapt it to individual situations. With growing surgical experience, each surgeon will develop his or her preferred approach to each technical problem.

[33]

The most innovative variation to the technique of vaginal hysterectomy was developed by Doderlein and Kronig in 1905 and was more recently described by Bohm in 1976 (15). This technique involves initial entry into the anterior cul-de-sac but not into the posterior pouch of Douglas. The bladder is elevated to allow the fundus of the uterus to be grasped and pulled into view. In the same sequence as a Heaney abdominal hysterectomy, the infundibulopelvic ligaments, uterine arteries, and cardinal ligaments are sequentially isolated and ligated. The uterosacral ligaments and posterior vagina are incorporated into the final pedicles to complete the hysterectomy. The author describes the successful application of this procedure in 285 patients and suggests that this technique has the advantage of reduced blood loss from early uterine vessel ligation and the absence of a posterior vaginal incision. This method was reportedly helpful in facilitating the transition from abdominal to vaginal hysterectomy in resident education programs.

Uterine destruction during vaginal hysterectomy

The greatest limitation to the surgeon's ability to routinely perform vaginal hysterectomy is uterine size. The most common indication for hysterectomy, uterine fibroids, is often associated with increased uterine size and is usually managed with an abdominal rather than a vaginal hysterectomy (6). Techniques to reduce uterine size intraoperatively and facilitate vaginal hysterectomy include uterine hemisection or bivalving, morcellation, and coring. All of these methods have been shown to be effective tools to safely aid in removal of the enlarged uterus.

Simple bivalving or hemisection of the uterus is helpful to increase exposure of the uterine fundus and improve access to the infundibulopelvic ligaments. A midline sagittal incision is made from the cervix to fundus after ligation of the uterine vessels. One half of the uterus is pushed aside to allow exposure of the remaining half. This simple technique is most applicable to uteri that are minimally enlarged and in which fundal exposure is modestly compromised. Significantly enlarged uteri often require more extensive destruction of the myometrium to accomplish vaginal hysterectomy.

In 1941, Lash popularized uterine coring as a method of removing 12–14 week-size uteri vaginally (16). Following ligation of the uterine arteries, a circumferential incision is made around the cervix, wide enough to encompass all of the endometrium and a majority of the myometrium. Traction is placed upon the cervix and this incision is progressively continued in a gradually widening cylindrical fashion up to the fundus. The incision should encompass the majority of the myometrium without breaching the serosal layer to leave behind a relatively thin shell of the uterus. This method was particularly recommended when vaginal hysterectomy was desired and a suspicion of endometrial carcinoma was present. Coring allowed the uterus to be safely debulked while leaving the endometrium intact.

The feasibility of vaginal hysterectomy with uterine coring was studied by Kovac in a retrospective review of a series of 902 hysterectomies (17). Vaginal hysterectomy was completed in 727 cases and the Lash coring technique was utilized in 76% of the vaginal hysterectomies. There was no significant difference in uterine weight between uteri removed abdominally (40–875 g) or by vaginal hysterectomy with coring (100–750 g). Uterine size in the simple vaginal hysterectomy group was significantly smaller than the other two groups. Mean operative time and length of stay was lower in both vaginal groups than the abdominal group and morbidity was similar across all groups. The author noted that the size of uterus removed by vaginal hysterectomy with coring increased as the surgeon's experience and comfort with the technique grew.

Wedge morcellation, or piecemeal removal of the uterus, is another method to allow vaginal removal of an enlarged uterus. Uterine morcellation can be accomplished in a variety of ways and can be tailored to the situation at hand. Initial hemisection of the uterus can be followed by removal of sections of myometrium, gradually moving medially to laterally. This is particularly appropriate when central fibroids are present. Alternatively, morcellation of the intact uterus can begin with removal of myometrium from the anterior or posterior walls, gradually moving toward the endometrium. Leiomyomata located in the superficial myometrium are removed as they are encountered using standard myomectomy techniques. Wedge resection of the uterus can also be performed by sequentially removing wedge-shaped sections of uterus beginning with the cervix and moving toward the fundus. The reduction in uterine bulk and width contributes to greatly improved exposure. Inherent to morcellation is destruction of the myometrium and the endometrial cavity with the possible spread of a uterine sarcoma or endometrial carcinoma. Prior to embarking upon a morcellation procedure, it is imperative that the endometrial cavity be adequately sampled in any patient at risk of carcinoma.

The decision to proceed to morcellation during vaginal hysterectomy will vary with the experience of the operator and will depend on uterine mobility, adhesions, location and size of fibroids, and space afforded by the vagina. The technical difficulty of these procedures mandates the use of two qualified surgical assistants. Pratt, in 1970, reviewed a personal series of 1512 vaginal hysterectomies and found an incidence of morcellation of 7.8% (18). He most commonly employed this technique in patients 36 to 60 years old and on uteri ranging from 66–700 gm. The mean size of the morcellated uteri was approximately 2 to 2.5 times larger than non-morcellated uteri. Perioperative morbidity was slightly higher in patients undergoing morcellation, but hospitalization stays and general outcomes were similar in both groups.

More recently, Grody reviewed a series of 324 consecutive vaginal hysterectomies of myomatous uteri over a 25-year period (19). The uteri ranged from 195–810 g, and all were removed by bivalving, coring, morcellation, or a combination of these techniques. Complications associated with destructive vaginal hysterectomy included five episodes of postoperative bleeding requiring surgical attention and four inadvertent cystotomies, which were all repaired without complication. The infec-

[35]

tious morbidity dropped from an initial rate of 16% to 10% following the initiation of routine antibiotic prophylaxis and a change to synthetic suture.

Destruction of the uterus by morcellation, coring, or bivalving allows the surgeon the opportunity to remove enlarged uteri vaginally and avoid the morbidity of an abdominal procedure. The literature suggests that these techniques are safe and feasible if applied in an individualized manner, taking into account the needs of the patient and the skill of the surgeon involved.

Concurrent ovarian removal

The decision to remove the ovaries at the time of hysterectomy is dependent upon ovarian function and accessibility. Oophorectomy is commonly performed in the postmenopausal patient to avoid reoperation for pathology and to reduce the risk of ovarian carcinoma. The place of oophorectomy in late reproductive age and perimenopausal women remains controversial as the actual reduction in cancer risk and the adequacy of hormone replacement remains unclear (20–22). Oophorectomy has been more commonly performed during abdominal hysterectomy than a vaginal hysterectomy—either due to oversight or limited access. Although technically more challenging, oophorectomy can and should be attempted during vaginal hysterectomy. The same indications for oophorectomy at abdominal hysterectomy should be applied to vaginal hysterectomy.

Smale has studied the feasibility and safety of salpingo-oophorectomy at the time of vaginal hysterectomy. Of 485 cases reported, oophorectomy was successful in 355 (73%) women (23). His technique involved incorporation of the fimbriated end of the fallopian tube into the utero-ovarian ligament pedicle. The infundibulopelvic ligament was then double-clamped and tied and the fallopian tube and ovary were then resected. Pathologic lesions, including a metastatic endometrial carcinoma, were present in 20% of the removed fallopian tubes and ovaries. Complications from concurrent salpingo-oophorectomy were limited to one laparotomy for infundibulopelvic ligament bleeding. Although retrospective and uncontrolled, this study suggests that salpingo-oophorectomy is feasible in many women undergoing vaginal hysterectomy and is associated with little additional morbidity.

Capen reviewed his experience with vaginal oophorectomy in 77 women undergoing hysterectomy (24). The method described differed from that of Smale. Prior to oophorectomy, the round ligament was isolated and ligated. A smaller pedicle can then be taken across the mesosalpinx to remove the fallopian tube and ovary, allowing a greater distance between the clamp and the ureter. Complications were limited to one reoperation due to bleeding from an infundibulopelvic ligament. The author found oophorectomy in the postmenopausal patient to often be technically more difficult due to shorter infundibulopelvic ligaments and estimated that 60–70% of ovaries could be removed through the vagina without difficulty.

[36]

The highest success rate of oophorectomy has been reported by Sheth (25). Of 1,440 women undergoing vaginal hysterectomy, oophorectomy was attempted in 740. Preoperative surgical indications, age, and parity were similar in both groups, and all women had a uterine size of less than 12 weeks. Oophorectomy was successful in 95% of cases and generally required 11–20 extra minutes of operating time. No complications could be attributed to the additional oophorectomy. Factors that increased the difficulty of oophorectomy included obesity, nulliparity, decreased vaginal access, lack of uterine mobility, inaccessible ovaries, and tubo-ovarian disease.

Limited mobility of the infundibulopelvic ligaments may be overcome by the use of an endoloop suture. Hoffman attempted oophorectomy at the time of vaginal hysterectomy in twenty patients ranging in age from 38–72 years (26). Oophorectomy was initially attempted in all patients using Capen's clamping technique. If standard oophorectomy was not feasible, removal was attempted by using an Ethicon 0 plain gut endoloop ligature. The ovary was grasped with a Babcock clamp and traction applied. The endoloop suture was then passed around the Babcock and secured on the mesovarium. A second endoloop suture was then placed close to the first and the ovary was excised under direct vision. Routine bilateral salpingo-oophorectomy was accomplished by the standard clamping technique in only four of 20 patients. Both ovaries were successfully removed in ten women using the endoloop technique after failure with clamp technique. One patient had bilateral oophorectomy using both techniques, and one patient had unilateral endoloop oophorectomy. In four patients, ovarian removal was impossible by either method. The author found the endloop method to require less operative space and afford better visualization of the mesovarium. This technique may be a feasible alternative to the standard clamping method of oophorectomy, particularly when ovarian mobility and visualization are limited.

Prophylaxis of vaginal vault prolapse

Genital prolapse following vaginal or abdominal hysterectomy can occur in 0.2–1.0% of patients (27). After completion of vaginal hysterectomy, attention must be turned to the repair and prophylaxis of any genital relaxation. Removal of the uterus without achieving adequate vaginal vault suspension provides little benefit to the patient and invites future prolapse.

The standard Heaney technique involves three steps for suspension of the vaginal apex (14). A suture is first passed through the anterior vaginal wall, then sequentially through the broad cardinal and uterosacral ligaments, and then the posterior vaginal wall on the ipsilateral side. This process is then repeated on the opposite side. Next, the uterosacral ligaments are plicated and finally the peritoneum is closed with a purse-string suture.

A modification of the Heaney technique was described by Cruikshank in 1987 (28). One hundred and twelve consecutive women underwent vaginal hysterectomy with attention to the vaginal vault to provide prophylaxis against posthysterectomy prolapse. After ligation of the uterosacral and cardinal ligaments, the pedicles were immediately sutured to the vaginal cuff. If the ligaments were lax, the pedicles were held until completion of the hysterectomy. When exposure was adequate, the lax ligaments were sufficiently shortened and then sutured to the cuff. In contrast to the Heaney technique, the broad ligaments were not sutured to the vaginal cuff. These relatively elastic vascular pedicles provide limited support to the vaginal apex and can be a source of deep dyspareunia. A purse-string suture was then placed using a 1-0 absorbable suture. In addition to encompassing the pedicles, the peritoneal suture was passed along the anterior rectal mucosa 3–4 cm above the peritoneal reflection to aid in obliteration of the posterior cul-de-sac and decrease the risk of future enterocele. Patients have been followed for 7 months to 3.5 years without evidence of posthysterectomy prolapse or enterocele.

Sacrospinous ligament suspension

Sacrospinous ligament fixation is a technique originally developed for repair of posthysterectomy vaginal vault eversion and has been well described by Morley and Delancey (29). Sacrospinous ligament fixation is accomplished by incising the posterior apex of the vagina and opening the pararectal space down to the right sacrospinous ligament. Sutures are then passed through the ligament, using caution to avoid the underlying neurovascular plexus, and attached to the serosal side of the vagina. As the vaginal mucosa is sutured closed, the sutures through the sacrospinous ligament are tightened to secure the vagina. Morley utilized this procedure in 71 patients with a 90% success rate. Of the remaining patients, 6% had good vault suspension but developed a symptomatic cystocele and 4% (three patients) failed the procedure.

Cruikshank has suggested that sacrospinous ligament fixation should be considered as an alternative method of preventing vault prolapse at the time of hysterectomy (30). Fixation of the uterosacral and cardinal ligaments to the vaginal vault may prevent future vaginal vault prolapse in the majority of patients but may not be adequate in patients with weak ligaments. Forty-eight women undergoing vaginal hysterectomy also had prophylactic sacrospinous ligament fixation performed. All were identified preoperatively to have uterovaginal prolapse and were found to have attenuated uterosacral and cardinal ligaments during hysterectomy such that vaginal cuff support would not be adequate. Morbidity from this additional procedure was limited to two episodes of bleeding from perirectal veins that required transfusion. Patients were followed for up to 3.2 years, and one episode of posthysterectomy vault prolapse was documented. This observational paper suggests that sacrospinous ligament fixation can be performed at the time of hysterectomy. However, the need to perform an additional procedure that does carry some associated morbidity must be weighed against the relatively low incidence of posthysterectomy vaginal vault prolapse. A prospective comparative trial of prophylactic sacrospinous ligament fixation and standard vault suspension techniques would address this question.

Enterocele repair

There are two classic approaches to repair of an enterocele at the time of vaginal hysterectomy: the McCall colporrhaphy and the Torpin wedge excision.

The McCall colporrhaphy involves obliteration of the hernial sac by placing a series of sutures from one uterosacral ligament across the redundant peritoneum to the opposite uterosacral ligament (31). The vaginal vault is then supported and suspended from the uterosacral ligaments by a series of two or three sutures sequentially passed through the posterior vaginal wall and both uterosacral ligaments. These plication sutures will securely attach the vaginal apex to the uterosacral ligaments and close off the enterocele space.

The Torpin wedge excision removes the enterocele by excision (32). A wedge-shaped section of vagina is excised between the uterosacral ligaments, and the full thickness of the defect is sutured together. The result is plication of the uterosacral ligaments, obliteration of the hernia site, and fixation of the vagina to the uterosacral ligaments.

Given retrospectively reviewed 68 cases of posterior culdoplasty performed over a 22-year period (33). Forty-eight were performed by the McCall culdoplasty technique and 20 cases by Torpin wedge resection of the cul-de-sac. Indications for culdoplasty included enterocele, procidentia, and complete vaginal vault prolapse after hysterectomy. The choice of procedure was made at the time of surgery. The Torpin method was used more often in older women with larger enteroceles in whom vaginal narrowing was not a great concern. Patients were followed for up to 20 years post-repair, with 30 patients who had McCall procedures and 17 who had Torpin procedures followed for five or more years. Two failures were identified, and both patients had been treated for complete procidentia with a McCall culdoplasty. Complications were few, with the notable exception of a ureteral obstruction in one patient with a McCall culdoplasy. Both of these methods of enterocele repair appear to be successful in this retrospective review. Further prospective analysis would be required to demonstrate a superiority of one method over the other.

Anterior and posterior colporrhaphy

Vaginal hysterectomy is accompanied by colporrhaphy in up to 44.5% of cases (6). Historically, anterior colporrhaphy has been indicated to reduce a symptomatic cystocele and provide treatment of mild to moderate genuine stress incontinence. Current literature has since documented the superiority of retropubic suspension techniques for management of stress incontinence. Posterior colporrhaphy remains the only means available for a rectocele repair. The current morbidity associated with these procedures is generally thought to be low. Dicker reviewed the mean duration of hospitalization for patients undergoing vaginal hysterectomy with and without colporrhaphy (6). Women undergoing additional colporrhaphy remained hospitalized an average of one day longer than standard vaginal hysterectomy. However, the five-day hospitalization associated with vaginal hysterectomy in 1981 is much longer than current standards. Taylor and Hansen compared the morbidity of anterior and posterior colporrhaphy in different age groups (34). The greatest morbidity was found in women under 35 years of age. Of 21 young women undergoing vaginal hysterectomy and colporrhaphy, 15 required blood transfusion, six developed a hematoma, and four developed a pelvic abscess. This increased morbidity among younger women was attributed to the increased pelvic vascularity of the reproductive age patient. No data was available on the degree of prolapse or difficulty of dissection in these patients. Anterior and posterior colporrhaphy are generally considered effective means of reduction of vaginal prolapse, although little current data is available to describe the morbidity associated with these procedures.

Peritoneal closure

The standard Heaney approach to vaginal hysterectomy calls for the placement of a peritoneal purse-string suture just prior to cuff closure. The rationale proposed for peritoneal closure includes extraperitoneal placement of pedicles to allow easier identification of postoperative bleeding, prevention of an intra-abdominal hematoma, and reduction in the incidence of posthysterectomy enterocele formation. As these goals can be achieved by uterosacral ligament plication and attachment of pedicles to the vaginal cuff during vaginal vault suspension, there is little value to this extra surgical step. A prospective randomized trial by Ling evaluated the feasibility of omitting peritoneal closure (35). Twenty-eight of 60 women undergoing vaginal hysterectomy were randomized to the no peritoneal closure group. No difference was present in operative indication, age, parity, or postoperative complications. In particular, the incidence of dyspareunia was similar in both groups. With little evidence of benefit to the patient, the practice of peritoneal closure during vaginal hysterectomy may be omitted.

Cuff closure

The best method of vaginal cuff closure has long been a source of debate among gynecologists. Various closure techniques vary from simple mucosal closure to combining cuff closure with vault suspension (36–38). Each method proclaims technical superiority, limited complications, and maintenance of a functional vaginal length. Few well-designed studies are available to adequately compare different methods of vaginal cuff closure.

Cruikshank prospectively compared five methods of vaginal cuff closure in 112 women (36). Following vaginal hysterectomy and vault suspension, the method of cuff closure was randomly assigned by sealed envelope. Five different techniques were utilized to evaluate the preservation of vaginal length and postoperative morbidity. Methods included

[40]

interrupted horizontal sutures, interrupted horizontal sutures placed laterally with running locked sutures centrally leaving a cuff opening, interrupted sutures placed longitudinally with running locked sutures in the lower one fourth of the cuff, continuous interlocking longitudinal sutures, and longitudinal interrupted sutures. In five patients, the randomly chosen closure was abandoned due to technical difficulties and the case was completed with a longitudinal closure. Vaginal depth was measured from the introitus to the anterior cervicovaginal junction before hysterectomy, at cuff closure, and at the six-week follow-up visit. Mean preoperative vaginal length for all patients in the horizontal closure groups was 10.1 cm and in the longitudinal closure groups, 10.4 cm. Vaginal lengths were not changed in either group immediately following surgery or at six weeks. No patient reported complaints of dyspareunia. Morbidity and complications were identical for all surgical groups. Either longitudinal or horizontal cuff closure can be used with equal success following vaginal hysterectomy.

Bladder catheter drainage after vaginal hysterectomy

The placement of a bladder catheter following vaginal hysterectomy is common practice. While affording some convenience to the surgeon to monitor fluid balance, catheterization does not provide any advantage to the patient. Summitt et al. prospectively randomized 100 women undergoing vaginal hysterectomy without colporrhaphy to catheterization for 24 hours postoperatively or no catheterization (39). Febrile morbidity and the postoperative incidence of urinary tract infection were compared between the two groups. Two patients in the catheter group and no patients in the no catheter group required recatheterization for the inability to void. Febrile morbidity was significantly higher in the catheterized patients (24.5%) than the no catheter group (8.0%) with one febrile episode directly attributed to a urinary tract infection in a catheterized patient. The incidence of urinary tract infection two days and two weeks postoperatively was not significantly different in either group. Avoiding bladder catheterization after vaginal hysterectomy decreases patient discomfort, allows early ambulation and same-day discharge, and reduces expense. Spontaneous voiding was not associated with any increase in urinary tract infections and may be associated with a decrease in overall febrile morbidity.

Vaginal packing following colporrhaphy

The placement of a gauze packing following vaginal plastic surgery is standard for many gynecologic surgeons. The development of fascial planes during an anterior or posterior colporrhaphy invariably causes interruption of small blood vessels, resulting in diffuse bleeding, and the placement of a vaginal pack achieves hemostasis by pressure on the raw surfaces. Two cases of retroperitoneal hematoma following vaginal hysterectomy with anterior and posterior colporrhaphy and vaginal packing were reported by Parulekar in 1989 (40). Both patients presented with vaginal bleeding and hemodynamic changes 6 to 8 hours postoperatively, and exploration revealed a retroperitoneal hematoma. Ligation of the anterior division of the internal iliac artery was required for hemostasis. Recognition of the hematoma may have been delayed by the presence of vaginal packing by allowing retroperitoneal spread rather than vaginal drainage. Although the placement of vaginal packing is routine for many surgeons, little data is available to evaluate the advantages or disadvantages of vaginal packing.

Additional complications of vaginal hysterectomy

In addition to the well-recognized complications of bleeding, infection, or recurrent prolapse associated with vaginal hysterectomy, the surgeon must also bear in mind the functional complications of vaginal surgery. Deep dyspareunia can result from midline plication of the ovarian pedicles or attachment of the ovaries to the vaginal cuff. Likewise, overzealous anterior or posterior colporrhaphy can significantly reduce vaginal capacity and form abnormal tissue ridges. The reduction of a large enterocele by a Torpin or McCall procedure can also significantly limit upper vaginal capacity. Careful preoperative attention to the patient's continued desire for sexual function is important to avoid these difficult-to-correct errors.

Summary

Lower morbidity and faster patient recovery make vaginal hysterectomy the procedure of choice whenever abdominal hysterectomy is not clearly indicated. New developments, such as laparoscopically assisted vaginal hysterectomy, combined with existing methods of uterine morcellation may now allow many larger uteri to be removed vaginally. Ongoing critical review of existing and developing surgical techniques will provide the gynecologic surgeon with a solid foundation on which to approach vaginal surgery.

References

1 Pokras R, Hufnagel VG. Hysterectomy in the United States, 1965–84. Am J Public Health 1988;78(7):852–853.
2 Barter RH. Vaginal hysterectomy. Clin Obstet Gynecol 1982;25(4):863–867.
3 Nichols DH. Vaginal versus abdominal hysterectomy. In: Stovall TG, ed. Current topics in obstetrics and gynecology—Hysterectomy. New York: Elsevier Science Publishing Company, 1993:27–33.
4 Leventhal ML, Lazarus ML. Total abdominal and vaginal hysterectomy: a comparison. Am J Obstet Gynecol 1951;61(2):289–299.
5 White SC, Wartel LJ, Wade ME. Comparison of abdominal and vaginal hysterectomies. Obstet Gynecol 1971;37(4):530–537.
6 Dicker RC, Greenspan JR, Strauss LT, et al. Complications of abdominal and vaginal hysterectomy among women of reproductive age in the United States: The Collaborative Review of Sterilization. Am J Obstet Gynecol 1982;144(7):841–848.
7 Stovall TG, Ling FW, Henry LC, Woodruff MR. A randomized trial evaluating leuprolide acetate before hysterectomy as treatment for leiomyomas. Am J Obstet Gynecol 1991;164(6):1420–1425.

[42]

8 Summitt RL Jr, Stovall TG, Lipscomb GH, Ling FW. Randomized comparison of laparoscopy-assisted vaginal hysterectomy with standard vaginal hysterectomy in an outpatient setting. Obstet Gynecol 1992;80(6):895–901.

9 Stovall TG, Summitt RL Jr, Bran DF, Ling FW. Outpatient vaginal hysterectomy: a pilot study. Obstet Gynecol 1992;80(1):145–149.

10 Lazar MR, Krieger HA. Blood loss in vaginal surgery: A comparative study. Obstet Gynecol 1959;13(6):707–710.

11 England GT, Randall HW, Graves WL. Impairment of tissue defenses by vasoconstrictors in vaginal hysterectomies. Obstet Gynecol 1983;61(3):271–274.

12 Cruikshank SH. Surgical method of identifying the ureters during total vaginal hysterectomy. Obstet Gynecol 1986;67(2):277–280.

13 Hofmeister FJ, Wolfgram RC. Methods of demonstrating measurement relationships between vaginal hysterectomy ligatures and the ureters. Am J Obstet Gynecol 1962;83(7):938–948.

14 Malpositions of the uterus. In: Mattingly RF, Thompson JD, eds. Te Linde's operative gynecology. Sixth edition. Philadelphia: J. B. Lippincott Company, 1985: 541–567.

15 Bohm JW, Lee FYL. Vaginal hysterectomy by anterior delivery of the uterine corpus. South Med J 1976;69(12):1543–1547.

16 Lash AF. A method for reducing the size of the uterus in vaginal hysterectomy. Am J Obstet Gynecol 1941;42:452–459.

17 Kovac SR. Intramyometrial coring as an adjunct to vaginal hysterectomy. Obstet Gynecol 1986;67(1):131–136.

18 Pratt JH, Gunnlaugsson GH. Vaginal hysterectomy by morcellation. Mayo Clin Proc 1970;45(5):374–387.

19 Grody MHT. Vaginal hysterectomy: the large uterus. J Gynecol Surg 1989;5(3): 301–312.

20 Tobacman JK, Tucker MA, Kase R, Greene MH, Costa J, Fraumeni JF Jr. Intra-abdominal carcinomatosis after prophylactic oophorectomy in ovarian-cancer-prone families. Lancet 1982;2:795–797.

21 Grogan RH. Reappraisal of residual ovaries. Am J Obstet Gynecol 97(1):124–129.

22 Counseller VS, Hunt W, Haigler FH Jr. Carcinoma of the ovary following hysterectomy. Am J Obstet Gynecol 1955;69(3):538–546.

23 Smale LE, Smale ML, Wilkening RL, Mundy CF, Ewing TL. Salpingo-oophorectomy at the time of vaginal hysterectomy. Am J Obstet Gynecol 1978;131(2):122–128.

24 Capen CV, Irwin H, Magrina J, Masterson BJ. Vaginal removal of the ovaries in association with vaginal hysterectomy. J Reprod Med 1983;28(9):589–591.

25 Sheth SS. The place of oophorectomy at vaginal hysterectomy. Br J Obstet Gynaecol 1991;98:662–666.

26 Hoffman MS. Transvaginal removal of ovaries with endoloop sutures at the time of transvaginal hysterectomy. Am J Obstet Gynecol 1991;165(2):407–408.

27 Symmonds RE, Williams TJ, Lee RA, Weeb MJ. Posthysterectomy enterocele and vaginal vault prolapse. Am Obstet Gynecol 1981;140(8):852–859.

28 Cruikshank SH. Preventing vault prolapse and enterocele after vaginal hysterectomy. South Med J 1988;81(5):594–596.

29 Morley GW, DeLancey JOL. Sacrospinous ligament fixation for eversion of the vagina. Am J Obstet Gynecol 1988;158(4):872–881.

30 Cruikshank SH, Cox DW. Sacrospinous ligament fixation at the time of transvaginal hysterectomy. Am J Obstet Gynecol 1990;162(6):1611–1619.

31 McCall ML. Posterior culdoplasty: Surgical correction of enterocele during vaginal hysterectomy; a preliminary report. Obstet Gynecol 1957;10(6):595–602.

32 Torpin R. Excision of the cul-de-sac of Douglas. J Intl College Surgeons 1955; XXIV(3):322–330.

33 Given FT Jr. Posterior culdoplasty: revisited. Am J Obstet Gynecol 1985;153(2): 135–139.

34 Taylor ES, Hansen RR. Morbidity following vaginal hysterectomy and colpoplasty. Obstet Gynecol 1961;17(3):346–348.

35 Ling FW, Stovall TG, Summit RJ Jr, et al. Peritoneal closure at the time of vaginal hysterectomy: a reassessment. Read at the Meeting of the Society of Gynecologic Surgeons, March 3, 1992, Orlando, Florida.

36 Cruikshank SH. Methods of vaginal cuff closure during vaginal hysterectomy. South Med J 1988;81(11):1375–1378.

37 Hajj SN. A simplified surgical technique for the treatment of the vault in vaginal hysterectomy. Am J Obstet Gynecol 1979;133(8):851–854.

38 Grossman RA. A new cuff closure technique for vaginal hysterectomy. Am J Gynecol Health 1988;II(3):30–32.

39 Summitt RL Jr, Stovall TG, Bran DF. Prospective comparison of indwelling bladder catheter drainage with no catheter after vaginal hysterectomy. Am J Obstet Gynecol 1994;170:1815–1821.

40 Parulekar SV. Posthysterectomy broad ligament haematoma: a complication of vaginal packing? J Postgraduate Med 1989;35(1):51–53.

4 Laparoscopically Assisted Vaginal Hysterectomy: Electrosurgical Techniques

D. ALAN JOHNS

Since the first laparoscopic hysterectomy was reported by Harry Reich in 1989 (1), laparoscopically assisted vaginal hysterectomy (LAVH) has become widely accepted as an integral part of gynecologic surgery. Despite this acceptance, there is little agreement among experts on the most efficient and cost-effective techniques for LAVH. The very existence of this book is a testament to this lack of consensus.

This chapter will outline:
• equipment necessary to complete LAVH using electrosurgical techniques,
• electrosurgical principles and tissue effects,
• laparoscopic techniques and principles required for successful completion of LAVH,
• when to consider LAVH,
• more importantly, when *not* to consider LAVH,
• when to start, and
• when to stop.

Simply stated, LAVH should offer patients the advantage of conversion from what would otherwise be an abdominal operation to a vaginal procedure. If this conversion is associated with minimal or no additional risk, shorter recovery, and costs no greater than abdominal hysterectomy, benefits are unquestionable.

Unfortunately, LAVH is often performed when vaginal hysterectomy is not only possible, but preferable. Prolonged operating times, expensive disposable equipment, and significant complications combine to make LAVH the "most expensive hysterectomy" (2,3). However, when good endoscopic skills are combined with adequate and inexpensive equipment, the properly selected patient will benefit with minimal additional risk.

Equipment

In most circumstances, a minimal amount of equipment is necessary to complete LAVH using electrosurgical techniques. Disposable equipment is expensive, offers little or no advantage, and should be avoided.

Ten- to 12-mm reusable trocars are used through the umbilical incision, the larger sleeve being necessary for use with the CO_2 laser. The larger visual channel of the 10-mm diagnostic laparoscope makes it the preferred endoscope for operative laparoscopy. Most LAVHs may be completed with two additional 5-mm suprapubic sleeves placed 3–6 cm on either side of the midline. Again, disposable trocars offer nothing but additional cost.

The various components of the video system comprise the surgeon's "eye" and are (arguably) the most important part of the operating room setup. With this in mind, every operating suite performing advanced operative laparoscopic procedures *must* be equipped with the best available combination of laparoscope, light source, videocamera, and monitor. To not have crisp, clear, true video images from which to work invites disaster.

A control system for suction/irrigation should be capable of delivering irrigation fluid through several different instruments (scissors, electrosurgical instruments, dissecting probes, graspers, etc.). Intermittent irrigation through these instruments helps maintain a clear operating field, allowing better identification of tissue planes. In addition, irrigation through electrosurgical instruments permits precise identification and control of bleeding vessels.

A non-electrolyte irrigation fluid, i.e., glycine (4), should be used. When passed through electrosurgical instruments, non-electrolyte solutions do not affect current flow, combining the benefits of constant irrigation with electrosurgery. Irrigation through these instruments during coaptation also limits lateral thermal injury and minimizes adherence of the bipolar blades to tissue. These solutions are considerably less expensive than isotonic or buffered electrolyte solutions.

Stapling devices must be passed through 12-mm trocars, increasing the risk of trocar injury to abdominal wall structures and postoperative fascial hernia. These staplers may be somewhat quicker but are very expensive and do not offer enough advantages over electrosurgical hemostasis to offset their cost. Stapling devices cannot be used when vascular pedicles have been dissected and skeletonized; they are simply applied across "wads" of tissue, providing hemostasis by compressing the tissue around the vessels.

Electrosurgical coaptation of vessel walls is most effective when the vessels have been isolated and skeletonized. Dissection does not significantly slow the surgery but minimizes risk of thermal injury to adjacent structures (5). When dense adhesions require careful dissection of structures before control of vessels, electrosurgery might be the safest and most efficient method of control. Furthermore, the large size of the stapling devices often precludes their use when large pelvic masses (myoma) must be removed. In these circumstances, the endoscopic surgeon must be proficient in endoscopic dissection and alternative methods for hemostasis.

The relationship between postoperative adhesion formation, sutures, staples, and energy sources is well documented (6,7,8). Postoperative adhesions are most likely to form when sutures or staples are used. Lasers and electrosurgery produce fewer postoperative adhesions. Regardless of the modality used for hemostasis, however, postoperative adhesions following LAVH are rarely a clinically significant problem.

The gynecologic laparoscopist *must* have available (and be familiar with) endoscopic suturing techniques. When bleeding occurs in proximity to vital structures, sutures may be the safest method for control. These endoscopic sutures must be immediately available to the surgeon. The operating room staff must be familiar with these sutures and be able to respond quickly and efficiently when brisk bleeding occurs.

Electrosurgical grasping forceps are mandatory items in the operating suite. Whether the surgeon prefers unipolar or bipolar electrosurgery, irrigation through these instruments during the desiccation process is important. This limits lateral thermal injury by cooling tissue next to the forcep blades and thereby minimizes the risk of thermal injury to adjacent structures. In addition, irrigation fluid cools the electrodes and minimizes adherence of desiccated tissue to the electrodes. If irrigation fluid cannot be passed through these instruments, the same effect may be obtained by constant irrigation of the area from a secondary probe.

The endoscopic surgeon *must* be experienced in dissection techniques. The safest vessel to coaptate is the one that has been dissected and isolated from surrounding tissue. Whether at laparotomy or laparoscopy, the pelvis "frozen" with adhesions or endometriosis requires careful dissection. The magnifying capability of the laparoscope gives the endoscopic surgeon an unequaled "close-up" view of the pelvis, allowing precise, careful dissection.

Laparoscopic dissection requires only two instruments—a blunt, hollow dissection/irrigation probe and a pair of reusable laparoscopic scissors with non-overlapping jaws. The more important requirement is a good working knowledge of pelvic anatomy. Injuries are not generally caused by instruments; they are caused by the instrument operator. Before attempting a difficult LAVH, the surgeon must be skilled in identification of pelvic structures and in dissecting and isolating these structures. This most often can be accomplished using simple blunt "aqua" dissection with either the dissection probe or closed scissors.

When electrosurgical energy sources are used, vessels should be dissected and isolated to effectively avoid undesired thermal injury. After most of the tissue surrounding the vessel has been removed, it is sealed (coaptated) with either unipolar or bipolar current. When the vessel walls have been desiccated while pressed together, adequate "weld strength" is attained to counteract either arterial or venous pressure (5,9,10). Sutures or staples are necessary only when bleeding follows inadequate coaptation.

Manipulation of the uterus will be necessary during the procedure. This is accomplished with a transcervical manipulator. Many large uteri, however, are impossible to move with an intrauterine manipulator. Strong grasping forceps with teeth may be useful in manipulating these large masses.

Electrosurgical considerations

A steady flow of electrons heats and dries (desiccates) the tissue through which it moves. Increasing the flow of electrons and using a noncontact electrode vaporizes (cuts) tissue. To seal a vessel, the surgeon must hold the vessel walls together while passing a flow of electrons through the tissue (9,10). If blood continues to flow through the vessel during the attempt at coaptation, energy is dissipated, and the vessel walls (which are not in apposition) will not "weld" together.

The vessel to be coaptated (sealed) must be occluded with electrosurgical forceps *before* current is applied. Both unipolar and bipolar instruments accomplish the desiccation equally well. In either instance, the flow of electrons slowly desiccates the vessel walls, "welding" them together.

Cutting current produces a steady flow of electrons through tissue with minimal wattage (11). This slow, steady current flow produces uniform desiccation of tissue. This concept is important since the goal is to uniformly desiccate all of the tissue between the forcep blades. When superficial tissue is quickly desiccated, it impedes the flow of electrons, preventing adequate desiccation of the deeper tissue. The result is incomplete desiccation, inadequate weld strength, and unwanted bleeding.

Although the surgeon might be able to visually determine the end point of vessel desiccation, a more objective and reproducible end point is more desirable. If bipolar techniques are used, an in-line ammeter tells the surgeon when current flow through tissue stops. At this point, tissue between the bipolar forcep blades should be thoroughly desiccated and vessels coaptated.

Bipolar current passes *only* through tissue between the blades of the bipolar forceps; it does *not* pass though distant areas or "arc" to adjacent tissue. The desiccation process, however, does produce heat that can damage adjacent structures. Slower coaptation with lower wattage helps to limit lateral thermal injury. Constant irrigation of the area with fluid also aids in cooling surrounding tissue, further limiting the risk of thermal injury.

To review, the risks associated with electrosurgical control of major vessels can be significantly decreased by:

1 careful identification and dissection of vessels to be controlled,
2 isolation of these vessels from surrounding structures,
3 utilization of bipolar cutting current,
4 use of an objective endpoint monitor to assess vessel wall desiccation,
5 irrigation of the tissue and bipolar forcep blades with a non-electrolyte solution to minimize lateral thermal injury,
6 a thorough knowledge of pelvic anatomy, and
7 familiarity with the physics and tissue effects of electrosurgical energy.

Other considerations

The gynecologic surgeon should *never* attempt LAVH without an extensive background and experience in operative laparoscopy. The patient requiring the laparoscopic approach to her hysterectomy is likely to have considerable pelvic pathology; otherwise, she would be a candidate for simple vaginal hysterectomy. If minimal or no pathology is found at laparoscopy, vaginal hysterectomy should be performed (12). For example, if the surgeon is planning a laparoscopically assisted vaginal hysterectomy in a patient with endometriosis, he (or she) should have extensive experience in the laparoscopic treatment (including excision) of endometriosis. Similarly, the gynecologist should have considerable experience with laparoscopic dissection of the pelvic sidewall before attempting the removal of ovaries during LAVH in the patient with severe adhesive disease.

The surgeon must gain skill, hand-eye coordination, and experience in simple laparoscopic procedures, e.g., salpingectomy, sterilization, etc., before progressing to more complex ones. Adenexectomy for benign disease, oophorocystectomy, treatment of extensive pelvic adhesive disease, and identification/dissection of the ureters should be well within the laparoscopic surgeon's capabilities before LAVH is attempted. The skills associated with these procedures are often required for safe completion of many laparoscopically assisted vaginal hysterectomies. Without these endoscopic skills, LAVH may be an exercise in frustration for the surgeon and a serious risk for the patient.

LAVH is *not* a substitute for a lack of skill in vaginal surgery. To complete LAVH in the patient who is truly not a candidate for vaginal hysterectomy, considerable skills in vaginal *and* laparoscopic surgery are required. If the surgeon is uncomfortable with the difficult vaginal hysterectomy, problems will be compounded during the difficult LAVH. Laparoscopic techniques simply allow completion of those portions of the procedure that would otherwise be impossible with a vaginal approach.

In addition, LAVH adds the risks associated with laparoscopy to those of hysterectomy (vaginal or abdominal). Complications of laparoscopic surgery, although uncommon, tend to be major (13,14,15). These complications include bowel perforation, major vessel injury, ureteral injury, and delayed bowel injury (usually thermal). None of these risks are commonly associated with abdominal or vaginal hysterectomy since neither of these procedures commonly requires a trocar. If these risks are to be added to those of hysterectomy, they must be offset by significant benefits to the patient.

The patient must be informed of the potential risks associated with laparoscopic surgery, regardless of the endoscopic procedure planned (16). The patient should agree that the potential advantages of the endoscopic approach to her hysterectomy is worth the risks associated with laparoscopy. The patient must make the decision to assume that added risk, not the doctor.

Patient selection

If a patient is to undergo hysterectomy for a benign process and would require an abdominal approach to complete her procedure, she would be a candidate for LAVH. Unfortunately, numerous variables make this simple rule extremely difficult to apply. There are as many indications and contraindications to vaginal hysterectomy as there are surgeons willing to compile them. One surgeon's contraindication to vaginal hysterectomy may be another's indication. This simply reflects a wide variance in skill and expertise in vaginal surgery.

Conversely, a surgeon may be skilled in vaginal surgery but very inexperienced in advanced endoscopic surgery techniques. This surgeon will be very skeptical of LAVH in those patients he or she feels cannot (or should not) undergo simple vaginal hysterectomy. These surgeons feel the hysterectomy that is too complex for a vaginal approach (in their hands) should not be approached with a laparoscope.

The surgeon who is very uncomfortable performing a vaginal hysterectomy (with or without removal of the ovaries) may see LAVH as a "crutch" for lack of skill in vaginal surgery. Rather than be something less than state of the art, this surgeon may turn what would otherwise be a 60–90 minute abdominal hysterectomy into a 3–5 hour surgical disaster.

The skilled "abdominal" surgeon may be able to perform a difficult abdominal hysterectomy more quickly and with fewer complications than if the same procedure were attempted laparoscopically. In the hands of this surgeon, the laparoscope may add little but problems.

LAVH should be undertaken by the gynecologic surgeon who is highly skilled in operative laparoscopy *and* vaginal surgery. Laparoscopic techniques should compliment the skills and abilities of the vaginal surgeon, thereby permitting completion of those portions of the operation that could not be performed vaginally. This could include excision of endometriosis, cul-de-sac dissection to allow colpotomy, adhesiolysis, ureteral identification and dissection, lysis of bowel adhesions, freeing of adhered adnexa, and control of infundibulopelvic vessels before vaginal hysterectomy.

Each gynecologic surgeon must honestly assess his or her skills in endoscopic, vaginal, and abdominal surgery. Under the appropriate circumstances, endoscopic techniques may allow a patient to enjoy the benefits of vaginal surgery with little additional risk. Most importantly, however, the route chosen to complete the hysterectomy must be cost-effective, maximize benefits, and minimize risks. This route to the pelvis will vary from one physician to another. It should never be determined by patient demand or the marketplace.

Further, LAVH is not a reasonable substitute for simple vaginal hysterectomy. Recent studies have shown LAVH to be more expensive than vaginal hysterectomy (17,18,19). LAVH also requires more operative time, more equipment, and more operating room personnel. It is likely, although not proven, that LAVH also adds significant risks to the relatively uncomplicated vaginal approach. To date, therefore, there is no justification for the use of endoscopy when simple vaginal hysterectomy is possible. In this circumstance, there are valid reasons to avoid the laparoscope.

Patient positioning

Inadequate positioning of the patient for laparoscopic surgery often precedes a very frustrating experience for the entire operating room. The patient must be optimally positioned for each portion of the procedure (endoscopic and vaginal). One position will *not* suffice for both. Operative laparoscopy requires the patient to be in the dorsal lithotomy position with both legs positioned low, the thigh level with the abdominal wall (Figure 4-1). Vaginal surgery requires the patient to be positioned with the legs high and lateral, allowing maximum room for the assistant to work.

When the position of the patient on the operating table causes the surgeon to struggle, time is lost and mistakes may occur. Begin the endoscopic portion of the operation with the patient in the optimum position for laparoscopic surgery. Once the endoscopic portion of the procedure is complete, take the time, usually no more than five minutes, to position the patient as you would for simple vaginal hysterectomy (Figure 4-2). This small investment in time will be offset by simplifying the vaginal portion of the LAVH.

Surgical technique

Since there are as many different techniques for hysterectomy as there are surgeons, endoscopic techniques for each step of the surgery will be reviewed separately. It is assumed the surgeon is (at least) familiar with laparoscopic equipment and electrosurgical principles as applied to endoscopy.

Identification and control of the ovarian vessels

It is always important to identify and isolate the ovarian artery and vein before using electrosurgical techniques for their control. This is easily accomplished from the retroperitoneal approach.

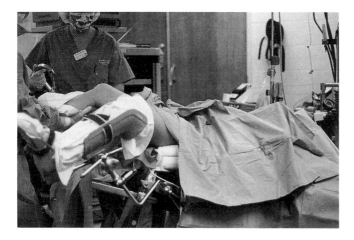

Figure 4-1 The dorsal lithotomy position.

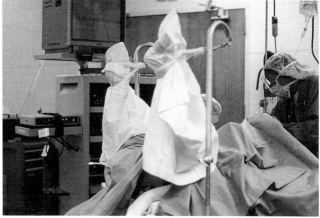

Figure 4-2 The patient is positioned as for vaginal hysterectomy, with legs high and lateral.

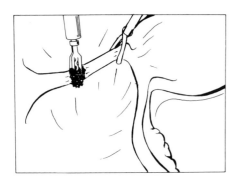

Figure 4-3 The round ligament is desiccated and transected.

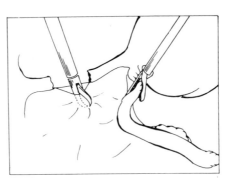

Figure 4-4 The peritoneal incision is extended between the round and infundipulopelvic ligaments.

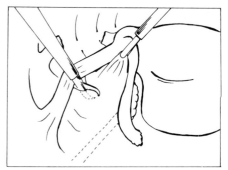

Figure 4-5 Peritoneam and connective tissue are dissected from the ovarian artery and vein.

The round ligament is desiccated and transected, permitting access to the retroperitoneal space (Figure 4-3). The peritoneal incision is extended between the round and infundibulopelvic ligaments with reusable scissors (Figure 4-4). The peritoneum is dissected away from pelvic sidewall structures, including the ureter, with a blunt dissection probe. This process is facilitated by fluid forced through the dissection probe, i.e., aquadissection. Peritoneum and connective tissue are carefully dissected from the ovarian artery and vein, isolating 2- 3-cm segments of these vessels in the process (Figure 4-5).

The ureter is carefully identified as it crosses the pelvic brim. After dissection, the skeletonized portions of the ovarian vessels should be isolated well away from the ureter and iliac vessels.

Bipolar cutting current is then passed through the skeletonized portions of the ovarian vessels with bipolar forceps (Figure 4-6). Adequate desiccation is evident by decreasing current flow measured by an ammeter. Constant irrigation of the area with a non-electrolyte solution will minimize lateral thermal injury and decrease the risk of injury to adjacent structures (ureter, iliac vessels).

If bleeding occurs after transection of the vessels, it is controlled by further desiccation or loop sutures. Prior skeletonization and dissection of the vessels greatly increase the ease with which this is accomplished.

Safe electrosurgical control of the ovarian vessels requires careful dissection and isolation of these vessels. Once this skill has been acquired, laparoscopic electrosurgical control of these vessels is as quick as stapling and much more precise.

After the ovarian artery and vein have been isolated, skeletonized, coaptated, and transected, the medial leaf of the broad ligament is opened with reusable laparoscopic scissors. This incision is carried parallel to the ureter to the uterine artery (Figure 4-7).

The pelvic sidewall dissection is then completed by dissection of retroperitoneal connective tissue and vessels away from the ureter and sidewall structures. The ovary and tube should now be completely freed from the pelvic sidewall and remain attached to the uterus.

If the adnexal structures are densely adherent to the pelvic sidewall, the retroperitoneal approach allows the peritoneum overlying the sidewall to be removed from lateral structures. The peritoneum is stripped from the sidewall with the ovary remaining attached. This technique should also decrease the risk of leaving behind an ovarian remnant.

Detachment of the ovary from the uterus

When clinical circumstances dictate retention of the ovary, electrosurgical techniques become somewhat more tedious and difficult. The large vessels in the broad ligament must be controlled at their attachment to the uterus. With patience, skill, and a good understanding of anatomy, however, electrosurgery may be used to accomplish this process.

The round ligament is desiccated and transected approximately 2–3 cm from its attachment to the uterine fundus. Using a blunt dissection/irrigation probe, vessels in the broad ligament are dissected medially and the medial leaf of the broad ligament is identified. The tube is desiccated at the uterotubal junction and transected. The utero-ovarian ligament is then identified, desiccated, and transected.

The medial leaf of the broad ligament is identified and opened. The remaining vessels in the broad ligament are desiccated and transected. The remaining peritoneum comprising the broad ligament is then opened to the uterine artery (Figure 4-8).

It is critical that the surgeon resist the temptation to grasp large portions of the broad ligament with bipolar forceps and attempt to desiccate these pedicles. When a large volume of tissue is grasped and desiccation attempted, most often vessels deep in these large pedicles are incompletely desiccated, and coaptation does not occur. The result may be bleeding from the large veins in the broad ligament that will be difficult to control.

Ureteral identification and dissection

Regardless of the techniques used for hemostasis, the ureters *must* be identified throughout their course in the pelvis. Positive identification will aid in dissection and avoid thermal or mechanical injury during the surgery. Not surprisingly, this rule has not changed since the beginning of

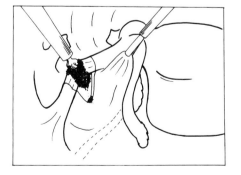

Figure 4-6 Biopolar current is passed through the skeletonized portions of the ovarian vessels.

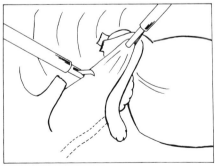

Figure 4-7 The medial leaf of the broad ligament is opened, and the incision carried parallel to the ureter and uterine artery.

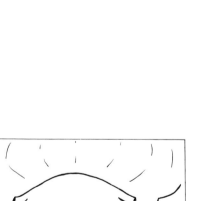

Figure 4-8 The remaining peritoneam comprising the broad ligament is opened to the uterine artery.

[53]

pelvic surgery. Unfortunately, endoscopic surgeons occasionally choose to ignore these basic surgical principles. Surgical access through small incisions should never negate these tenants of surgery.

The ureters are most easily identified as they cross the pelvic brim. From this point, their course may be followed by direct transperitoneal visualization or dissection, depending on clinical circumstances. If the ureter is not visible or readily apparent, it must be positively identified. If this requires dissection of the retroperitoneal space, it should be done. The endoscopic surgeon must be prepared to take whatever means necessary to identify the ureters, including laparotomy.

Conversely, it is not always necessary to dissect the ureters throughout their course in the pelvis. Simple visual identification of these structures next to critical areas will most often suffice.

The uterine artery

Most gynecologists with some expertise in vaginal surgery are very comfortable controlling the uterine artery vaginally. It is a rare patient in which the surgeon is unable to safely place a clamp across the cardinal ligament, including the uterine artery, transvaginally. Since ureteral injury commonly occurs at the level of the uterine artery, common sense would dictate the surgeon should use those techniques most familiar to him or her to avoid such injuries.

On the basis of preoperative examination, if the surgeon determines the uterine arteries must be controlled endoscopically, careful dissection and isolation of these vessels will permit their safe electrosurgical coaptation. Laparoscopic suturing may also be effective but requires considerable skill and patience.

The uterine artery can easily be identified by careful blunt dissection after the broad ligament has been opened. All connective tissue must be removed and the uterine vessels dissected away from the ureters and pelvic sidewall. Only when 1–2 cm of the vessel are isolated should electrosurgery or sutures be utilized for control.

Prior to its bifurcation into the uterine and cervical branches, the isolated segment of the uterine artery is coaptated with bipolar cutting current. The bipolar forcep is placed next to the uterus, just as a clamp would be placed during vaginal or abdominal hysterectomy. After transection, the surgeon may choose to place a loop suture around the proximal stump of the uterine artery. Remember, constant irrigation of the portion of the artery undergoing coaptation will limit lateral thermal injury.

Because of the proximity of the ureter, the uterine artery *must* be identified, skeletonized, and isolated before any attempt is made to control the vessel. If this cannot be accomplished, or if the uterine artery cannot be identified, the laparoscopic portion of the procedure should be abandoned. In the vast majority of cases, there is no need to attempt control of the uterine artery endoscopically. This step is more easily and safely performed during the vaginal portion of the procedure.

The cardinal and uterosacral ligaments

As with the uterine artery, transection of the cardinal and uterosacral ligaments is rarely essential to complete the hysterectomy vaginally. When necessary, the cardinal ligament is isolated from the pelvic sidewall, desiccated, and transected. Desiccation can be accomplished using bipolar or unipolar electrosurgery. It will be helpful to incise the peritoneum overlying these ligaments prior to desiccation. A unipolar needle using cutting current will also transect these structures easily. Bleeding is controlled with fulguration (coagulation current applied with the active electrode off tissue) or bipolar desiccation.

Because the cardinal and uterosacral ligaments are thick, thorough desiccation is difficult. The process will produce considerable thermal injury to the surrounding tissues. For this reason, cutting of these structures with the unipolar needle is often preferable. A clean cut is produced with minimal bleeding and minimal thermal injury when the needle is properly used. This requires adequate wattage, a small needle, and a nontouch technique. The uterus and lower uterine segment must be retracted away from the pelvic sidewall to safely accomplish this step utilizing electrosurgery.

Before the uterosacral ligaments are transected, the rectum should be dissected well away from the area. This requires an incision into the peritoneum overlying the cul-de-sac between the uterosacral ligaments. This incision should be at the junction of the uterosacral ligaments and lower uterine segment. Dissection of the rectum away from the posterior vagina and rectovaginal septum is easily accomplished with a blunt dissection/irrigation probe.

Endoscopic completion of this step will isolate the rectum from the uterosacral ligaments and lessen the chances of rectal injury. In addition, posterior colpotomy will be easier, should that step be required.

The bladder

Opening the peritoneum overlying the vesicouterine fold and dissection of the bladder from the anterior lower uterine segment facilitates the vaginal portion of the operation and should be considered in most cases.

The peritoneum is grasped and lifted as the uterus is pushed cephalad with the uterine manipulator. The peritoneum will be stretched, allowing the surgeon to better identify the vesicouterine junction. An incision is made in the peritoneum with reusable laparoscopic scissors or unipolar electrosurgery (Figure 4-9).

The proper plane is identified between the bladder and lower uterine segment and the bladder is dissected away using a blunt dissection/irrigation probe and aquadissection. Once the proper plane is identified, this dissection is quick, easy, and relatively bloodless. The bladder is dissected laterally to the cervical branch of the uterine artery. Continuous traction on the bladder coupled with cephalad pressure on the uterus greatly facilitates this dissection.

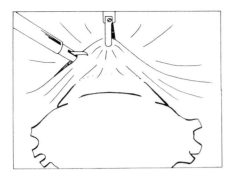

Colpotomy

When unusual circumstances require the entire hysterectomy to be completed by laparoscopic techniques, anterior and posterior colpotomy will be necessary. As previously stated, dissection of the rectum away from the posterior vagina and cervix simplifies posterior colpotomy.

A tenaculum placed on the posterior lip of the cervix is used to apply traction while the cul-de-sac is distended with a moist sponge. The cul-de-sac should be readily identifiable endoscopically. The rectum should be well away from this area, and the uterosacral ligaments transected.

An incision is made in the posterior cul-de-sac with a unipolar needle using cutting current. Once the cervix is identified, the incision is extended around both sides of the cervix to the anterior cul-de-sac. Bleeding is controlled with spray fulguration (nontouch fulguration with coagulation mode current).

The bladder has been previously dissected away from the anterior lower uterine segment, allowing identification of the anterior cul-de-sac. This is achieved by distending the vagina above the cervix with a moist sponge. Unipolar electrosurgery is the most efficient method for opening the vagina anteriorly. Again, fulguration is used to control bleeding.

The uterus and adnexal structures are now free and can be removed by fragmentation or morcellation. The vaginal cuff may be closed endoscopically or vaginally, depending on clinical circumstances. The method requiring the shortest operative time should be chosen.

Reinspection

After the vaginal cuff has been closed, the pneumoperitoneum is reestablished and the operative field inspected. Bleeding is controlled with electrosurgery (usually bipolar). Occasionally, large vessel bleeding is discovered. This occurs most often when large myomatous uteri must be morcellated and removed by fragmentation. As large fragments are removed, they are pulled over coaptated vessels, occasionally opening those vessels. These bleeding vessels are controlled with bipolar desiccation or sutures, depending on their location.

Clots may conceal venous bleeding and should be removed. Underlying vessels can be inspected and fulgurated as necessary. All major vessel pedicles are carefully inspected. Clots and debris are removed by copious irrigation. If the integrity of the ureters is in question, they are catheterized and inspected. As the final step, the upper abdominal cavity is inspected for abnormalities or injury.

Discussion

The advantages of vaginal over abdominal hysterectomy is unquestioned. The ability of laparoscopic techniques to allow vaginal hysterectomy when the abdominal approach would otherwise be necessary is also obvious. What remains is to determine the safest and most cost-effective method for converting abdominal to vaginal hysterectomy.

Several studies have addressed the indications for and safety of
LAVH (13,14,16,19). Serious complications associated with LAVH have
also been reported (14). Since there is no standardized definition for
laparoscopically assisted vaginal hysterectomy, a staging system (21) has
been devised to accurately describe the extent of the endoscopic portion
of the hysterectomy (Table 4-1). It is hoped that this staging system will
allow accurate comparisons of LAVH between institutions and investigators. In addition, the endoscopic portion of the procedure most likely to
result in complications may also be identified. This data, which is yet to
be published, may indicate the safest endoscopic method for converting
abdominal to vaginal hysterectomy.

Considering the current economics of health care, the most cost-
effective method for LAVH must also be determined. It is unlikely, although unproven, that disposable laparoscopic equipment offers any economic advantage over reusables. Do other methods of hemostasis, e.g.,
clips, staples, etc., offer advantages adequate to overcome their cost? Do
they significantly shorten operative time? Are they safer than electrosurgery? Are they associated with fewer immediate post-operative and
long-term problems? Can they be disposed of in an ecologically sound
manner? These questions must be answered before the electrosurgery
versus staples debate is over.

Most likely, there is no correct method. Circumstances encountered
in the operating room should dictate the safest and most cost-effective
method for completing the operation.

The endoscopic surgeon should become proficient in the use of both
electrosurgery and stapling devices. The cost of disposable devices, as
well as reusables, used in each case should be known to every surgeon in
every operating suite. Furthermore, the laparoscopic surgeon should be
aware of the total costs associated with each procedure performed. The
benefits and risks of each modality can then be intelligently ascertained.

With the health care crisis looming everywhere, it is mandatory that
gynecologic surgeons carefully evaluate every procedure from all stand-

Table 4-1 Laparoscopically assisted vaginal hysterectomy (LAVH) staging

Stage

0—Laparoscopy done—No laparoscopic procedure performed prior to vaginal hysterectomy
1—Procedure included laparoscopic adhesiolysis and/or excision of endometriosis
2—Either or both adnexa freed laparoscopically
3—Bladder dissected from uterus
4—Uterine artery transected laparoscopically
5—Anterior and/or posterior colpotomy or entire uterus freed
SUBSCRIPT:
    0—Neither ovary excised
    1—One ovary excised
    2—Both ovaries excised

NOTE—If the extent of the procedure performed laparoscopically varied on the
right and left pelvic sidewalls, stage the procedure by the most advanced side. (Reproduced with permission from Johns DA, Diamond MP. Laparoscopically assisted
vaginal hysterectomies. J Reprod Med 1994;39:424–428.)

points. Are there more cost-effective alternatives to surgery? When surgery is necessary, what is the safest and most cost-effective method for completion of that surgery? With respect to LAVH, time and experience will answer these questions.

References

1 Reich H, DeCaprio J, McGlynn F. Laparoscopic hysterectomy. J Gynecol Surg 1989;5:213–226.

2 Baggish MS. The most expensive hysterectomy. J Gynecol Surg 1992;8:57–58.

3 Boike GM, Elfstrand EP, Del Priore G, Schumock D, Holley HS, Lurain JR. Laparoscopically assisted vaginal hysterectomy in a university hospital: report of 82 cases and comparison with abdominal and vaginal hysterectomy. Am J Obstet Gynecol 1993;168(6, Part I):1690–1701.

4 Soderstrom RM. Glycine as an irrigant during microsurgical hemostasis. A microsurgeon's observations. J Reprod Med 1991;36(4):256–265.

5 Ryder RM, Hulka JF. Bladder and bowel injury after electrodesiccation with Kleppinger bipolar forceps. A clinicopathologic study. J Reprod Med 1993;38(8):595–598.

6 Grainger DA, Meyer WR, DeCherney AH, Diamond MP. Laparoscopic clips. evaluation of absorbable clips and titanium with regard to hemostasis and tissue reactivity. J Reprod Med 1991;36(7):493–495.

7 Luciano AA, Maier DB. Electrosurgery and lasers in endoscopic pelvic surgery. Infertil Reprod Med Clin NA 1993;4(2):255–274.

8 Guerre EF Jr., Diamond MP. Adhesions prevention: Does anything work? Infertil Reprod Med Clin NA 1993;4(2):275–288.

9 Harrison JD, Morris DL. Does bipolar electrocoagulation time effect vessel weld strength? Gut 1991;32:188–190.

10 Dunn MR, Sigel B. The mechanism of blood vessel closure by high frequency electrocoagulation. Surg Gynecol Obstet 1965;823–831.

11 Odell RC. Electrosurgery in laparoscopy. Infertil Reprod Med Clin NA 1993;4(2):289–304.

12 Kovac SR, Cruikshank SH, Retto HF. Laparoscopy assisted vaginal hysterectomy. J Gynecol Surg 1990;6:185–193.

13 Davis GD, Wolgamott G, Moon J. Laparoscopically assisted vaginal hysterectomy as definitive therapy for Stage III and IV endometriosis. J Reprod Med 1993;38(8):577–581.

14 Lee CL, Soong YK. Laparoscopic hysterectomy with Endo GIA 30 stapler. J Reprod Med 1993;38(8):582–586.

15 Woodland MB. Ureter injury during laparoscopy assisted vaginal hysterectomy with the endoscopic linear stapler. Am J Obstet Gynecol 1992;167(3):756–757.

16 Phipps JH, John M, Hassanaien M, Saeed M. Laparoscopic and laparoscopically assisted vaginal hysterectomy: a series of 114 cases. Gynaecol Endoscopy 1993;3:7–12.

17 Donovan JF, Van Voohis BJ. Legal issues in operative laparoscopy. Contemp Obstet Gynecol 1993;38(8):31–39.

18 Nezhat F, Nezhat C, Gordon S, Wilkins E. Laparoscopic versus abdominal hysterectomy. Journal Reprod Med 1992;37(1):247–250.

19 Boike GM, Efstrand EP, Laurain JR. Laparoscopically assisted vaginal hysterectomy in a university hospital: report of 50 cases with comparison to vaginal and abdominal hysterectomy. Presented at the Central Association of Obstetricians and Gynecologists, Chicago, Illinois November, 1992.

20 Summitt RL Jr, Stovall TG, Lipscomb GH, Ling FW. Randomized comparison of laparoscopy assisted vaginal hysterectomy with standard vaginal hysterectomy in an outpatient setting. Obstet Gynecol 1993;80(6):895–901.

21 Johns DA, Diamond MP. Laparoscopically assisted vaginal hysterectomies. J Reprod Med 1994;39:424–428.

5 Laparoscopically Assisted Vaginal Hysterectomy: Stapling Technique

BRYAN R. KURTZ

Laparoscopically assisted vaginal hysterectomy (LAVH) has quickly become a procedure at the forefront of gynecology, promoted by surgeons who view it as a viable alternative to abdominal hysterectomy, and rapidly growing in acceptance by a patient population interested in minimally invasive health care. Indeed, LAVH is often compared to laparoscopic cholecystectomy, a procedure that rapidly grew in popularity due to patient demand. However, just as laparoscopic cholecystectomy has sparked controversy in the field of general surgery, the growth in LAVH has led to considerable debate as to its proper role in what is considered standard care.

Proponents of LAVH tout the procedure as a reasonable alternative to abdominal hysterectomy, with the benefits of decreased postoperative pain and hospitalization as well as faster return to routine activities (1–5). In our practice, we have found a high degree of patient satisfaction with the procedure (5). Opponents of the procedure express concern that overzealous and undertrained surgeons may perform the procedure on patients who could have simply undergone a cheaper and quicker vaginal hysterectomy. While this may be true in some circumstances, certain patients in our practice now can avoid laparotomies. We have found that the procedure requires a combination of competent skills in both endoscopic and vaginal surgery. Our LAVH experiences have actually increased our skills in vaginal surgery, and, therefore, our selection criteria for patients who are candidates for vaginal hysterectomy has expanded. This phenomenon seems to be especially true in our residency program, where, traditionally, there has been weak training in vaginal hysterectomy.

This chapter will discuss the technique of LAVH using stapling devices. At our institution, we had the opportunity to perform preclinical trials on these devices. As LAVH caught on in our community, the majority of surgeons started to use these devices. Although we have gradually converted to the use of electrosurgical techniques for our cases, the majority of our staff continue to prefer the stapling devices, due to simplicity and traditional concerns over the safety of electrosurgery. However, with increased education on the principles of safe electrosurgery, this trend may change. It is an interesting phenomenon that so many gynecologic surgeons have so quickly embraced the use of stapling devices, when, with the exception of gynecologic oncologists, they have little or no previous experience with surgical stapling techniques. This reflects the successful aggressive marketing activities of stapling manufacturers. This chapter will focus on the development and utilization of stapling techniques for LAVH.

Principles of surgical stapling

Surgical stapling was demonstrated and first applied as early as 1908 (6). The principle then, as it is now, was first to gently compress and mobilize tissues followed by placement of the staples. From the start, the importance of using fine wire staples and placing double staggered rows for greater safety as well as the paramount principle of the B-closure of the staples was understood. Although staple shape has never been questioned, some later devices used coarser staples (7,8). Subsequently, however, all developers of stapling instruments have reverted to using the finer wire staples with double staggered rows.

Many of the refinements in surgical stapling devices are attributed to the intense efforts of the Scientific Research Institute for Experimental Surgical Apparatus and Instruments in Russia. A wide spectrum of problems relating to stapling was addressed, including tissue thickness, healing, metal use for the instruments and staples, and instrument design. New applications, not only to the gastrointestinal tract, including broncho-pulmonary structures, vessels, and even bones were developed (9). The Russian technology was brought to the United States in 1958 by Ravitch (10). Subsequent intensive engineering research and advances in technical concepts in both the U.S.S.R. and the United States combined with the availability of lighter strong metals and molded plastics has led to substantial refinements in instrument design and in operative surgical principles. The first generation of American-made instruments appeared in the late 1960s. These instruments incorporated many important advances, including the placement of all moving parts into the cartridge, transforming the instrument into a simple shell available for multiple uses, and the concept of disposable pre-loaded sterilized cartridges. Today, the instruments are represented by a family of staplers, including TA, GIA, EEA, LDS, and skin and fascia staplers, the first two of which have been adapted to laparoscopic use.

The TA instrument (U.S. Surgical, Norwalk, CT) places a double line of staggered staples without a means of transection. The TL instrument (Ethicon Endo-Surgery, Cincinnati, OH) is a competitive product, with similar design. Instruments are available in different lengths as well as staple sizes. Staple size, defined as leg length, is an important factor based on tissue thickness. These instruments are extensively used for closure of all portions of the gastrointestinal tract, although the most important use is in the various techniques for sealing pulmonary parenchyma prior to incision or excision. Recently, a TA stapler has been developed that uses an absorbable staple, Polysorb 55 lactomer co-polymer. This device has been used for abdominal hysterectomy since concern over proximity to vagina or urinary tract has prohibited the use of steel wire staples (11).

The GIA instrument (U.S. Surgical, Norwalk, CT) places two double staggered rows of staples and, in the same operation, divides the tissue between the two pairs of staggered rows. The instrument was originally designed to achieve anatomic side to side, minimally inverting, serosa to serosa anastomosis by placing each GIA limb into the lumen of the organ to be anastomosed. The residual opening is then either closed with sutures or with a mucosa to mucosa TA closure. Anastomoses from the esophagus to the rectum are performed with the GIA instrument. The TLC (Ethicon Endo-Surgery, Cincinnati, OH) is a similar competitive instrument.

Laparoscopic stapling devices

The first instrument adapted to laparoscopic use was the Multifire Endo-GIA, developed by U.S. Surgical Corporation (Figure 5-1). This device is a reloadable, mechanical stapling and cutting instrument, which places three rows of titanium staples on either side of a transection line. Two cartridges are available for the device. The white cartridge (30-V) uses staples with a leg length of 2.5 mm (Figure 5-2). After firing the instrument, the staples close to 1.0 mm, giving a tight closure, which is recommended for use on vascular structures. The blue cartridge (3.5) uses a staple with a leg length of 3.5 mm, which closes to 1.5 mm (Figure 5-3). The staple line in both of these cartridges extends approximately 34 mm. The knife blade transects the tissue at a length of approximately 29 mm. The Multifire Endo-GIA requires a 12-mm trocar to insert laparoscopically.

Recently, the U.S. Surgical Corporation has released the Multifire Endo-TA instrument (Figure 5-4). This instrument fires three rows of titanium staples, and there is no transection of the tissue. This instrument has the advantage of a narrower stapler line, about 6 mm in width. However, it still requires a 12-mm trocar.

Until recently, the U.S. Surgical Corporation has had a monopoly

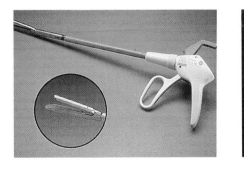

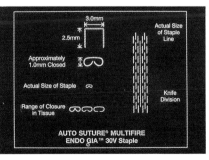

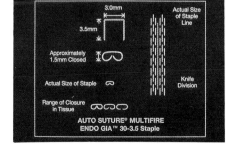

Figure 5-1 Endo-GIA instrument (U.S. Surgical, Norwalk, CT) with blue 3.5 cartridge.

Figure 5-2 Staple configuration for Endo-GIA 30-V staple.

Figure 5-3 Staple configuration for Endo-GIA 3.5 staple.

[61]

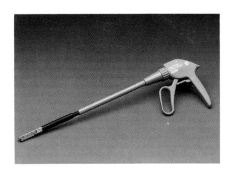

Figure 5-4 U.S. Surgical Endo-TA instrument with blue 3.5 cartridge.

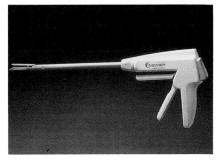

Figure 5-5 Endoscopic Linear Cutter (ELC) instrument (Ethicon Endo-Surgery, Cincinnati, OH) with blue 3.5 cartridge.

on the laparoscopic stapling market. However, Ethicon Endo-Surgery recently released their version of a laparoscopic stapling device, called the Endoscopic Linear Cutter (ELC) (Figure 5-5). The product has a reloadable cartridge that places staples with a 3.5-mm leg length that closes to 1.5 mm, similar to the Endo-GIA. We are presently performing preclinical trials on their vascular cartridge, which, similar to the Multifire Endo-GIA, has a 2.5-mm leg length, closing down to 1.0 mm. The ELC staple line is longer than the Endo-GIA, measuring approximately 38 mm (Figure 5-6). The transection line is also longer, measuring approximately 33 mm. Whereas the Multifire Endo-GIA is approved for four firings per staple gun, the ELC is approved for eight firings. This fact, combined with the longer staple length, may prove this instrument to be more cost effective than the Multifire Endo-GIA.

Indications for LAVH

As mentioned previously, LAVH is a procedure that is meant to replace abdominal hysterectomy. The decision to proceed with LAVH over vaginal hysterectomy is dependent upon the surgeon's expertise and comfort level with a vaginal approach. Similarly, the decision between LAVH and abdominal hysterectomy is dependent on the operator's skills in

Figure 5-6 Comparison of staple and cut lines for ELC-35 and Endo-GIA 30 staplers.

Table 5-1 Indications for LAVH

1 Pelvic pain, especially noncyclical
2 Known or suspected pelvic endometriosis
3 Significant uterine enlargement, i.e., fibroids
4 Previous pelvic surgery, including cesarean section
5 Acute or chronic pelvic inflammatory disease
6 Known or suspected pelvic adhesions
7 Known or suspected ovarian pathology
8 Minimal uterine descensus

both endoscopic and vaginal surgery. Potential indications for LAVH are listed in Table 5-1.

Surgical technique

After induction of adequate general anesthesia, the patient is placed in the dorsolithotomy position. The ability to easily change the position of the legs between the laparoscopic and vaginal portions of the procedure is imperative. Candy cane or shepherd hook stirrups are useful, although they may cause problems with stabilization of the knee. Allen stirrups provide stable support for the legs and can be easily raised or lowered, depending on the portion of the procedure. Care must be taken to avoid compression of the calf, thus placing all pressure on the heel of the foot.

Although a three-puncture technique has been described utilizing 12-mm trocars in the umbilicus and laterally, we prefer a four-puncture technique, adding a 5-mm trocar suprapubically to assist in dissection. Figure 5-7 demonstrates trocar placement. The lateral trocars should be placed fairly high to give a proper angle for directing the stapling device across the infundibulopelvic ligaments if the ovaries are to be removed.

After initial inspection of the abdominal cavity, a decision is made to proceed with LAVH. The course of both ureters can be visualized in the majority of patients. The necessity for ureteral dissection prior to the treatment of vascular pedicles is controversial. We do not routinely dissect out the ureter, unless there is significant distortion of the pelvis from adhesions or endometriosis. Ureteral identification, however, is mandatory.

If the ovaries are to be removed, traumatic graspers are used to elevate and pull the tube and ovary medially to expose the infundibulo-pelvic ligament. A vascular stapling cartridge is then placed across the infundibulopelvic ligament (Figure 5-8). Occasionally, the round ligament can be incorporated in this initial bite, saving some time in the procedure. Another stapling device can be placed across the round ligament and upper broad ligament (Figure 5-9). Since the round ligament can sometimes be significantly thickened, a nonvascular cartridge may be more appropriate. U.S. Surgical Corporation has a gauging device that may be of assistance in choosing between a vascular and nonvascular cartridge. In order to save some money by reducing staple use, we will often merely bipolar coagulate the round ligament and

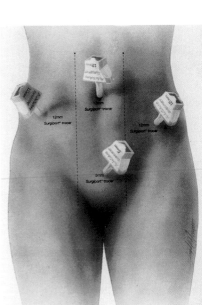

Figure 5-7 Four-puncture trocar placement for laparoscopically assisted vaginal hysterectomy.

[63]

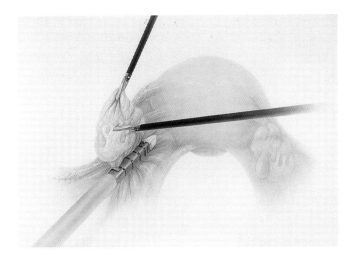

Figure 5-8 Placement of vascular stapler across the infundibulopelvic ligament.

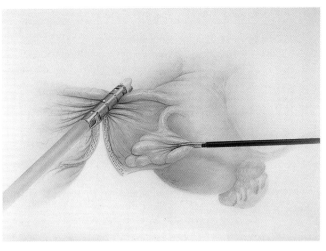

Figure 5-9 Placement of second stapler across the round ligament and upper broad ligament.

transect it sharply with scissors. Following transection of the round ligament, the upper broad ligament is usually fairly avascular.

If the ovaries are to be conserved, a stapling device can be placed across the proximal round and uterovarian ligaments. Again, this tissue can sometimes be thickened, and the nonvascular cartridge may be preferred. Occasionally, we will coagulate and transect the round ligament, and then place the stapler across the uterovarian ligament.

The next step involves incision of the vesicouterine peritoneum and dissection of the bladder from the lower uterine segment and cervix (Figure 5-10). We will usually make a small hole in the midline, and use aquadissection to elevate the peritoneum. The incision is then extended laterally using scissors, unipolar electrode, or laser energy. We feel that use of laser for LAVH is not indicated, since in our hospital, it adds significant cost to the procedure. The incision is extended to the staple

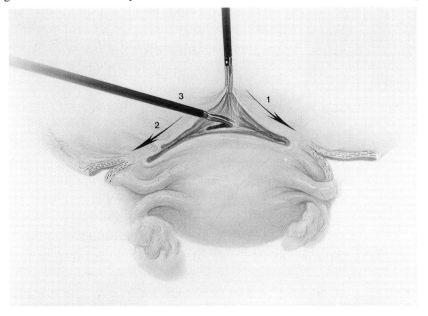

Figure 5-10 Incision of the vesicouterine peritoneum and dissection of the bladder from the lower uterine segment and cervix.

[64]

line at the upper broad ligament. The end of the staple line needs to be opened, which can be done sharply with scissors. It is recommended to avoid the use of unipolar coagulation near the staple line, as energy may be conducted down the staples, resulting in coagulation of the transected tissue.

Once the vesicouterine peritoneum is incised, the bladder is taken down with sharp and/or blunt dissection. A 5-mm laparoscopic pusher is a helpful instrument in dissecting the bladder. Unipolar or bipolar coagulation can be used to ensure hemostasis at the bladder pillars before transection. The uterine vessels are then skeletonized anteriorly. It is best to keep the posterior peritoneum in place over the uterine vessels so that the staples have a surface to which they can attach. To avoid ureteral injury, it is imperative that the bladder be taken down well below the internal cervical os and dissected laterally to allow the ureter to fall away from the cervix.

At this point, a decision should be made as to whether to clamp the uterine vessels laparoscopically or vaginally. We often find that it is easier to convert to the vaginal portion prior to transection of the uterine vessels so that we can clamp and suture them. If vaginal exposure is inadequate and we feel that we will not be able to get the uterine vessels vaginally, they can be stapled laparoscopically. It should be remembered, however, that the ureter is approximately 2 to 2½ cm away from the lateral cervix, running just underneath the uterine vessels. The stapling cartridge itself is approximately 12 mm in diameter. If the bladder is taken down adequately and the vessels are skeletonized anteriorly to allow the ureter to fall away, the vessels can be stapled safely. To ensure that we place the staples tightly against the lateral cervix, we will place the stapler through the umbilical trocar, using the lateral trocars to visualize with the laparoscope.

The Multifire Endo-TA instrument is especially useful to occlude the uterine vessels. Since it is narrower than the Endo-GIA, there is less concern about occluding the ureters, as long as the stapler is placed tightly along the lateral cervix. After a staple line is placed on each side, the tissue is transected sharply with scissors along the cervix.

It is not recommended that staplers be placed any lower than the upper cardinal ligament. Placement of staples across the lower cardinal or uterosacral ligaments may be too close to the vagina. There is concern that this may result in, or at least be implicated in, postoperative dyspareunia.

Once the decision is made to convert to the vaginal approach, we will proceed with colpotomy incision laparoscopically if visualization is adequate. A moistened sponge stick is first placed in the posterior vaginal fornix, and the bulging cul-de-sac is incised with unipolar coagulation. If descensus is still poor, we will occasionally transect the uterosacral ligaments at this point. We prefer to take these ligaments vaginally, however, so that we can ensure that they are adequately sutured into the vagina for pelvic support. After the posterior colpotomy incision is made, the uterus is dropped posteriorly to occlude the pneumoperitoneum. The moistened sponge stick is then placed in the anterior vaginal fornix, and, after ensur-

[65]

ing that the bladder is well down below the level of the vagina, we will open up the anterior cul-de-sac in a similar fashion.

The hysterectomy is then completed vaginally. A weighted retractor is placed through the posterior colpotomy incision, and a right-angle retractor is placed through the anterior colpotomy incision. The remainder of the cervix is then circumcised, and the lateral vagina is bluntly dissected off of the cervix. The uterosacral ligaments are clamped, incised, and tied off. We will incorporate the uterosacral ligaments into the lateral vagina. If the uterine vessels were previously transected laparoscopically, it is usually one more bite of tissue to free the lateral attachments of the uterus. Usually, the clamp must be placed with the assistance of a finger at the upper level of the remaining pedicle. This avoids placing the clamp inside of the previous transection line, resulting in redundant dissection. If the uterine vessels were not treated laparoscopically, we will take a third bite to clamp them. We will usually clamp both sides, then transect the tissue to free the uterus. The vessels are doubly ligated and the uterus is then removed through the vaginal cuff. If the uterus is significantly enlarged with fibroids, morcellation, either laparoscopically or vaginally, may be required.

The peritoneum is not closed as is done with routine vaginal hysterectomy. This is so that the pedicles can be examined laparoscopically after completion of the vaginal portion. We close the vaginal cuff in a running longitudinal fashion. We do not routinely place a vaginal pack, thus minimizing the patient's postoperative discomfort.

Laparoscopy is repeated to examine the pedicles. Hemostasis is achieved as needed with careful bipolar coagulation. Because of the elevated intraperitoneal pressure during laparoscopy, some bleeding may not be readily apparent. It is recommended that the pedicles be examined either under water or with reduced intraperitoneal pressure. The stapled pedicles should be examined in particular. The staples are not meant to necrose tissue, so there may be some oozing from the staple line. This can be controlled with bipolar coagulation. Again, monopolar energy should be avoided around the staple line, since energy may be transmitted across the staples. Once hemostasis is confirmed, we will often leave 200 to 300 cc of heparinized irrigation fluid within the pelvis to, hopefully, minimize postoperative adhesion formation. We use lactated Ringer's as an irrigation solution, as it has buffering capability, thus reducing the drop in pH any absorbed CO_2 may cause.

Advantages of LAVH

When compared to abdominal hysterectomy, several advantages of LAVH are apparent. The majority of our patients are discharged from the hospital within 24 to 48 hours following surgery. Some surgeons are actually performing LAVH on an outpatient basis with patients going home the same day. While in the hospital, we find our patients use less pain medicine and have quicker return of bowel function. Following discharge, the majority of our patients return to full activities, such as work or exercise, within two to three weeks. We have them refrain from intercourse for a full six weeks, however, due to healing of the vaginal cuff. We have found a high degree of patient satisfaction with the procedure (5). Furthermore, studies suggest decreased postoperative adhesion formation following laparoscopy compared to laparotomy (12).

Advantages of stapling devices for LAVH

Laparoscopic stapling devices offer a rapid hemostatic method of occluding and transecting tissue to perform LAVH. In our retrospective review of the initial experience of surgeons in our area, we found a significant savings in time between laparoscopic stapling devices versus bipolar coagulation (5). The average operating time for the stapling devices was one hour and 57 minutes compared to three hours and 43 minutes in initial procedures performed with bipolar coagulation. Subsequently, with experience and confidence, our operative times for LAVH using electrosurgical techniques have fallen to only two hours. Furthermore, by avoiding electrocoagulating current, many surgeons feel the stapling devices are safer near vital structures, such as the ureter. This fact remains to be proven, however, since there have already been reports of incidental stapling of the ureter with these devices (13).

Disadvantages of LAVH

As stated previously, LAVH is a procedure that requires advanced skills in both operative laparoscopy and vaginal surgery. Concern has been expressed that some surgeons may use LAVH on patients who should be vaginal hysterectomy candidates. This exposes the patient to unnecessary added costs and risks of complication from the laparoscopic portion of the procedure. Whereas retrospective reviews have demonstrated some cost saving over abdominal hysterectomy, a prospective study has shown no benefit of LAVH over vaginal hysterectomy in patients who are candidates for the latter (14). These investigators did note significant increase in costs to the patient undergoing LAVH.

Disadvantages of stapling devices for LAVH

Laparoscopic stapling devices require a 12-mm trocar for placement. This increases the risk to the patient of bleeding complications from laceration of the inferior epigastric vessel or from bleeding of the rectus muscle. To avoid this potential complication, it is imperative to attempt to visualize the inferior epigastric vessels and to try to place the trocar lateral to the rectus muscle. There have also been reports of incisional hernia through a 12-mm trocar (15). We routinely close the fascia with a figure-eight suture prior to closure of the skin incision at any trocar site greater than 10 mm.

The most significant disadvantage of the use of stapling devices as well as use of disposable instruments and trocars in general is the added cost to the procedure. We found that use of disposable instruments for

[67]

LAVH results in a $2,000 to $3,000 increase in costs. Much of the added cost is due to hospital markup. We were able to negotiate a reduction in markup for the disposable instruments for LAVH. However, with current changes in the health care system, hospital markup may no longer be an issue. If procedures are reimbursed at a set rate regardless of equipment used, then the hospitals will have to look at ways to cut their own costs. Perhaps without adding the markups to the cost of the stapling devices, the savings in OR time may help demonstrate these devices as a cost-effective alternative. The introduction of competition into the laparoscopic stapling market may also help drive down costs. The ELC produced by Ethicon Endo-Surgery can be fired more times than the Endo-GIA and will reportedly cost less. If the number of staplers used during the procedure is minimized and reusable instruments such as trocars and scissors are used, the staplers may prove cost effective. The best approach will probably be individualized for each case, using a combination of staplers and/or bipolar coagulation.

Conclusion

Just as laparoscopic cholecystectomy was for the general surgeons, LAVH is felt to be an important procedure in the field of gynecologic surgery. Its proper role in the armamentarium of the surgeon is yet to be completely defined. The fact that LAVH is not meant to replace vaginal hysterectomy is well established. Prospective studies are needed to confirm the advantages of LAVH over abdominal hysterectomy to properly define its role. The debate between laparoscopic stapling devices and bipolar coagulation will continue. However, now competition in the market and changes in health care reimbursement may equalize the cost differential between the two methods.

References

1 Reich H, DeCaprio J, McGlynnis F. Laparoscopic hysterectomy. J Gynecol Surg 1989;5:213–216.
2 Kovac S, Cruikshank S, Retto H. Laparoscopy assisted vaginal hysterectomy. J Gynecol Surg 1990;6:185–188.
3 Minelli L, Angiolillo M, Caione C, et al. Laparoscopically assisted vaginal hysterectomy. Endoscopy 1991;23:64–66.
4 Liu CY. Laparoscopic hysterectomy: a review of 72 cases. J Reprod Med 1992;37:351–354.
5 Daniell JF, Kurtz BR, McTavish G, et al. Laparoscopically assisted vaginal hysterectomy: the initial Nashville experience. J Reprod Med 1993;38:537–542.
6 Hültl H. II Kongress der Ungarischen Gesellschaft fur Chirurgie, Budapest, May 1908. Pester Med Chir Presse 1909;45:108–110,121–122.
7 von Petz A. Zur Technik der Magenresektion. Ein neuer Magen-Darnmähapparat. Zentralbl Chir 1924;51:179–188.
8 Friedrich H. Ein neuer Magen-Darm-Nähapparat. Zentralbl Chir 1934;61:504–506.
9 Steichen FM, Ravitch MM. Contemporary stapling instruments and basic mechanical suture techniques. In: Ravitch MM, Steichen FM, eds. The surgical clinics of North America, symposeum on stapling techniques. Vol. 3, Philadelphia, WB Saunders, 1984:425–440.
10 Ravitch MM, Brown IW, Daviglus GF. Experimental and clinical use of the Soviet bronchus stapling instrument. Surgery 1959;46:97–102.

11 Beresford JM. Automatic stapling techniques in abdominal hysterectomy. In: Ravitch MM, Steichn FM, eds. The surgical clinics of North America, symposium on stapling techniques. Vol. 3. Philadelphia: W. B. Saunders, 1984:609–618.

12 Diamond MP, Daniell JF, Johns DA, et al. Postoperative adhesion development after operative laparoscopy: evaluation at early second-look procedures. Fertil Steril 1991;55:700–704.

13 Woodland MB. Ureter injury during laparoscopy assisted vaginal hysterectomy with the endoscopic linear stapler. Am J Obstet Gynecol 1992;167:756–757.

14 Summitt RL, Stoval TG, Lipscomb GH, Ling FW. Randomized comparison of laparoscopy assisted vaginal hysterectomy with standard vaginal hysterectomy in an outpatient setting. Obstet Gynecol 1992;80:895–901.

15 Kurtz BR, Daniell JF, Spaw AT. An incarcerated incisional hernia following laparoscopy: a case report. J Reprod Med 1993;38:643–645.

6 Laparoscopic Hysterectomy by the Suture Method

LESLIE A. SHARPE

Hysterectomy is a common surgical procedure which has traditionally required laparotomy with its consequent pain and disability in 70 to 75% of all cases. Vaginal hysterectomy, a less invasive and less morbid alternative, has traditionally been done in 25 to 30% of all cases. Advanced laparoscopic surgical techniques have the potential to revolutionize the approach to hysterectomy, and to bring to many patients the benefits of minimally invasive treatment. Advanced suturing and knot-tying skills are key elements in this laparoscopic surgical revolution.

The greatest patient benefit occurs when abdominal hysterectomy is avoided, not when vaginal hysterectomy is replaced. Laparoscopic hysterectomy and laparoscopically assisted vaginal hysterectomy (LAVH) may be expected to increase steadily as laparoscopic technique and technology advance together. Suturing and knot-tying skills are necessary for the laparoscopic surgeon to achieve maximal conversion of abdominal hysterectomy to less invasive treatment.

Laparoscopy is not a procedure; it is merely another means of visualization. The procedure performed should be the same whether viewed on a video monitor or through a laparotomy incision. Expediency should not lead the surgeon to accept for laparoscopy any method that would be judged inadequate for laparotomy. Abdominal hysterectomy poses anatomical challenges in tissue repair that are best met by suturing. The laparoscopic approach must achieve comparable results if it is to be justified.

Laparoscopic suturing and knot tying have been relatively neglected because of their perceived difficulty. Other methods and ingenious mechanical devices have been substituted with varying degrees of success. In the author's opinion, recent improvements in technique and instrumentation have made the suture method simple, efficient, rapid, and reliable. The potential scope of laparoscopy is thereby greatly increased.

Suturing and knot-tying skills enable the laparoscopic surgeon to perform the entire hysterectomy procedure by a technique essentially identical to the traditional abdominal hysterectomy, without need of vaginal exposure or a large laparotomy incision. Laparoscopic hysterectomy is an alternative to abdominal hysterectomy in many cases where poor vaginal exposure contraindicates vaginal hysterectomy or LAVH. Related reparative procedures, such as retropubic urethropexy and vaginal vault suspension, may be done in addition to laparoscopic hysterectomy or LAVH by proven suture methods. The suture method extends the therapeutic range of operative laparoscopy and increases indications for its application in the hysterectomy procedure.

Patient selection

The availability of laparoscopy does not alter the accepted indications for hysterectomy or the diagnostic and nonsurgical methods to be applied before surgery is recommended. Given adequate surgical indications, laparoscopy may be appropriate if the pathology is within the scope of current instrumentation and technique and if the patient gives fully informed consent to attempted minimally invasive treatment.

Contraindications to laparoscopic treatment include the following:

1 Patient is unable to tolerate pneumoperitoneum or the table tilting necessary for exposure (example: hiatus hernia).

2 Severe adhesions prevent adequate access port placement.

3 Magnitude of the pathology exceeds the capability of the surgeon or the technique (examples: malignancy, pelvic cavity filled by mass too large to work around).

4 Adequate specimen retrieval is not feasible (example: ovarian cystic neoplasm too large for the available containment pouch, which would allow decompression without spillage into the peritoneal cavity).

5 Prompt appropriate response to complications is not feasible. Laparoscopic dissection in hazardous areas should not be done without the capability for instantaneous conversion to laparotomy.

Procedure planning

The preferred method of hysterectomy will depend upon the pathology present, the size of tissue masses to be removed, the possible need of a containment pouch to prevent spillage of infected or neoplastic tissues, the reparative procedures that will be necessary, and the presence of complicating features, such as obesity or adhesions. The procedure undertaken must address all of these concerns and provide a clearly planned method to deal with them.

After due consideration, the surgeon may conclude that laparoscopy is inappropriate due to malignancy or other severe problems. Abdominal hysterectomy is then the prudent choice. When the chosen method of hysterectomy proves difficult or complicated, the prudent surgeon may conclude that continuation is inappropriate and will, therefore, convert to abdominal hysterectomy.

After consideration, the surgeon may conclude that laparoscopy is unnecessary. Vaginal hysterectomy remains the preferred treatment when uterine size is relatively normal, vaginal exposure is adequate, and uterine attachments are all accessible; vaginal repair may be indicated also, and in such cases vaginal hysterectomy is usually feasible. Laparoscopy is of no benefit to any patient who may be managed by straightforward vaginal hysterectomy. The highly skilled vaginal surgeon may even be able to remove a significantly enlarged uterus by morcellation from below, accepting increased blood loss in order to avoid abdominal incision.

Regardless of the surgeon's skill, there are technical limits to the application of vaginal hysterectomy. The technical limits of vaginal hysterectomy are defined by the appearance of a number of negative factors: prolonged operating time, increased blood loss from the uterus until all vessels are secured, vaginal trauma due to prolonged forceful retraction, increased risk of infection due to repeated entry of the pelvic cavity through the contaminated vagina, and risk of collateral organ damage due to poor surgical exposure. At the limits of vaginal hysterectomy, either laparoscopy or abdominal hysterectomy becomes preferable.

LAVH requires sufficient vaginal exposure to allow management of the lower uterine attachments and the uterine arteries and sufficient laparoscopic exposure to manage the upper uterine and adnexal attachments. Morcellation, if needed, is generally done vaginally, followed by suturing of the vaginal cuff from below. The laparoscopic portion of LAVH may vary greatly from patient to patient and need be only enough to facilitate transvaginal completion of the procedure.

At the technical limits of LAVH, either laparoscopy will be unable to free the upper uterine attachments or vaginal exposure is inadequate for safe management of the lower attachments. When inadequate vaginal exposure is the limiting factor, laparoscopic hysterectomy remains available as an alternative to abdominal hysterectomy in selected cases.

Laparoscopic hysterectomy done by the suture method follows closely the internal steps of traditional abdominal hysterectomy. Vascular supply and ligamentous supports are suture ligated and cut free, then the specimen is morcellated laparoscopically as needed before removal through the vagina or a minilaporotomy incision. The vagina may be closed by suturing laparoscopically or vaginally at the surgeon's option. Subtotal hysterectomy may be done in selected cases when cervical pathology has been ruled out.

The technical limits of laparoscopic hysterectomy do not involve vaginal dimensions or cervical support, but rather the pelvic pathology, the size of the uterus, and the amount of pelvic exposure available for laparoscopic operation. Uterine enlargement to 20 weeks' pregnancy size usually does not prevent laparoscopic access to the adnexal attachments. A few centimeters of free space along the pelvic sidewalls is usually sufficient to allow identification of the ureters and suture ligation of the uterine arteries. The devascularized uterus may be amputated from the cervix to yield excellent exposure for the remainder of the procedure. Laparoscopic morcellation of the amputated fundus is bloodless. Adnexal masses up to 10-cm size may be freed intact and then placed in a containment pouch for decompression and morcellation without intraperitoneal spillage. Future technological advances in specimen management may be expected to extend even further the limits of laparoscopic hysterectomy as an alternative to abdominal hysterectomy.

A skilled laparoscopic surgeon may be unable to predict with certainty whether a patient may be treated safely by laparoscopic hysterectomy or require abdominal hysterectomy instead. Exploratory laparoscopy may be done to assess the patient and to initiate laparoscopic hysterectomy, if appropriate. As long as progress is satisfactory and the next step in the procedure may be taken safely, laparoscopic hysterectomy continues. If progress is stymied, the procedure is converted to abdominal hysterectomy with full benefit of the dissection already completed; a smaller incision may then be feasible.

A similar uncertainty may occur when deciding upon vaginal hysterectomy versus LAVH. It may be appropriate to begin with the vaginal portion of the procedure and to proceed as long as there is good progress and hemostasis. In some cases, the entire procedure may be completed as a vaginal hysterectomy, thus avoiding the extra expense of laparoscopy. If laparoscopy is, indeed, necessary, the vagina may be blocked with a vaginal access port (VAP) or a large wet pack to maintain pneumoperitoneum. The laparoscopic portion of the procedure may then be expected to be straightforward and readily able to identify the previously established planes of dissection.

Clearly, a great deal of thought must be given to modern hysterectomy planning. The surgeon must be aware of his or her skill level and the anatomical findings that will determine success or failure of a given approach. Growing mastery of laparoscopy techniques, including the suture method, may be expected to yield a steady increase in the utilization of laparoscopic hysterectomy and LAVH, with a parallel decline in abdominal hysterectomy. The surgeon who masters laparoscopic suturing will have the greatest flexibility in hysterectomy procedure planning.

Basic principles of the suture method

Access ports must be compatible with the passage of suture and able to maintain pneumoperitoneum when suture is present in the gas seal. Ball valve and trumpet valve access ports tend to cut suture and should not be used. Ports with a rubber flap or trapdoor-type gas seal are generally most suitable. Ports should be secured in place by suturing to the abdominal skin or by other mechanical means so that knot-tying and suturing maneuvers do not dislodge them. The greatest flexibility and speed in suturing are achieved when the needle in use will fit through any port in use; size 10–11 ports are most useful with the stout curved needles favored in gynecology. Use of large ports also allows movement of the laparoscope as needed for better view.

Extracorporeal knot tying using a closed-tip knot pusher allows the surgeon to maintain through it continuous control of one suture strand, place securely a double throw surgeon's knot with flat orientation, linear forces across the knot, and control precisely knot tension. Additional square knots are formed externally by one-handed technique, rapidly carried internally by the knot pusher, and tied as firmly as desired for knot security. This method is most frequently used by the author. It is powerful, flexible, and precisely controllable. The typical series of knots may be completed within 60 seconds.

Intracorporeal knot tying is enhanced if the swaged-on needle is retained as an aid to knot tying. When the tip end of the needle is grasped by a powerful needle holder, the heel end of the needle may be used to wrap loops of suture around an assisting instrument well away from its tip. The loops are thus more easily retained in position as the grasping instrument picks up the free end of suture and pulls it through the loops to form a knot. Knot tension is limited by the strength of the grasping instrument and the strength of swage of suture into the needle. This method is usually applied on relatively delicate tissues where maximum tension is not necessary.

Laparoscopic suturing during the author's hysterectomy procedure is done with a powerful needle holder having vertically oriented vise-like jaws capable of holding needles or sutures securely. Flat-sided curved needles work best, as they readily orient upright in the jaws and are then resistant to twisting or slipping. A 32-mm, ⅜ circle, flat-sided taper-point needle (Ethicon EN-2), swaged onto 36 inches of size 0 synthetic absorbable suture is suitable for use in hysterectomy.

The needle is readily introduced into the abdomen by grasping suture 1–2 cm away from it with the needle holder and then passing it through the access port (Figure 6-1). Once inside the abdomen, the needle must be oriented correctly for the intended stitch before it is loaded into the needle holder. The needle is first stabilized by grasping its tip end with a laparoscopic instrument, and then the needle is rotated in that instrument into proper position by pulling on the suture with the needle holder (Plate 1). Once the needle has been oriented to the intended direction of rotation, it is loaded into the needle holder. The stitch is placed with care to follow the proper plane of rotation through the tissues. To avoid twisting of the needle, it is helpful to stabilize its tip with a grasping instrument before it is released from the needle holder (Plate 2). The needle may then be pulled through the tissue without difficulty. The needle is retrieved from the peritoneal cavity by grasping suture 1–2 cm away from it with the needle holder, which then pulls it back out through the access port (Plate 3). The gas seal must be held

Figure 6-1 Needle holder grasps suture near needle to pull it heel-first through access port.

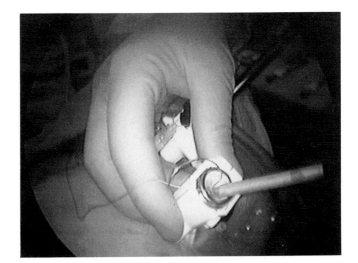

open as the needle passes through it in order to avoid jamming (Figure 6-2). Each stitch placed by this technique requires less than 60 seconds to complete.

Continuous suturing is done by repeating the above, using care to avoid entanglement of slack suture along the way. Slack is most easily managed when it is kept outside the body, where tangling is readily avoided. After each completed stitch, the needle is fully withdrawn through the access port, and all slack suture is pulled through the tissues. The assistant follows the continuous suture line by grasping the internal portion of the suture with an instrument, to keep it taut and out of the way as each succeeding stitch is made by the surgeon. At the end point of the continuous suture line, a second stitch is placed and tied to leave one strand long. After the continuous suture line has been completed, it is secured in place by tying to this long strand.

Laparoscopic suturing is most efficient when the surgeon carefully plans ahead the optimal direction of the needle rotation through the tissues, which port will allow proper orientation of the needle holder to achieve such needle rotation, and which port to insert the assisting instrument through, so that the stitch may be placed and the needle retrieved without crossing instruments or losing control of the needle.

A loaded needle holder is potentially dangerous and, therefore, must be kept in view at all times. Particularly when performing intracorporeal knot tying, the surgeon should ensure that the needle is clear of tissue before using it to apply force to the suture.

Optimal video imaging is critical to success in suturing where fine needle tips and suture strands must be discerned from surrounding tissues. A high-resolution camera and monitor, and an alert assistant who maintains a sharply focused upright view of the surgical field, must be coordinated closely with the surgeon's movements to enable success. Video monitor placement at the foot of the operating table allows both the surgeon and the assistant to work with the same well-oriented view of the surgical field.

Other apparatus is positioned off the head of the table so that the surgeon and assistant are not entrapped by hoses or wires and may change sides as needed to work on each side of the uterus. Changing sides helps to avoid awkwardness and reaching across the table. It is also helpful for the surgeon to be able to change hands and function ambidextrously as much as possible.

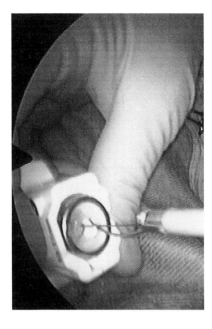

Figure 6-2 Gas seal is held open by surgeon as needle holder pulls needle heel-first through access port.

Instrumentation

A high-resolution video system is required for clear view of suture and needles. An automatic CO_2 insufflator with 9–15 L/min flow capacity is advisable to compensate for unavoidable gas losses while suture is handled through access ports. Access ports with ball valve or trumpet style gas seals should not be used, as they tend to snag and cut suture. Access ports having a trap door or rubber flap type gas seal are compatible with

[75]

manipulation of suture. Size 10–11 ports in all locations will allow most flexibility in use of a stout curved needle (Ethicon EN-2), which is advantageous during hysterectomy.

Operating speed is enhanced by use of 10-mm size hand instruments in order to avoid as much as possible the need to use down-sizing adaptors during exchange of instruments. The larger, more sturdy instruments also provide additional strength and utility during the hysterectomy procedure. The author's laparoscopic instrument set usually includes one extracorporeal knot pusher, one ligature carrier, one needle holder, two hemostats, two atraumatic forceps (one of which is used to hold a small cotton pledget inside a sponge aspiration device), one cutting dissector, and one VAP. If morcellation is required, two tenaculi are used to stabilize the tissue, which is cut by a spring-retractable scalpel for speed and safety (Figure 6-3).

The harmonic scalpel (UltraCision Corporation, Smithfield, RI) is used in well-vascularized tissues for its coagulating and cutting properties. The argon beam coagulator (ABC) (Birtcher Medical Systems, Irvine, CA) is used to control surface bleeding not managed by other measures. Monopolar electrosurgery is also useful, though accompanied by troublesome smoke generation. Irrigation is done directly through an

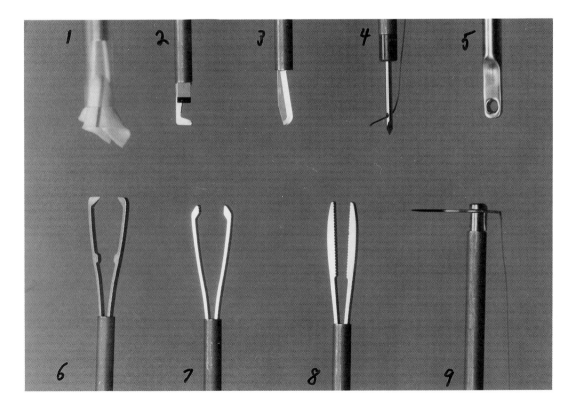

Figure 6-3 Instruments for hysterectomy: (1) sponge aspirator for suction, tamponade, and blunt dissection with 1½ inch square sponge loaded into it, (2) cutting dissector with powerful guillotine-type action, (3) scalpel with spring-retractable blade for safety in use, (4) ligature carrier with spring-retractable needle for safety in use, (5) knot pusher with closed tip to speed knot formation and prevent suture disengagement during knot placement, (6) tenaculum for grasp of solid tissue masses, (7) atraumatic forceps for non-crushing grasp of ureter, fallopian tube, or ligated pedicles, (8) hemostat for needle manipulation and powerful tissue grasp, and (9) needle holder with vertical jaws and vise-like grip on flat-sided needle (Ethicon EN-2). (Instruments courtesy of Sharpe Endosurgical Corporation, Minneapolis, MN.)

access port with a bulb syringe; the fluid is promptly evacuated with the sponge aspirator to maintain a clean field without troublesome pooling of irrigant.

Surgical technique

The patient is anesthetized, the trachea is intubated, and a nasogastric suction tube is placed. The legs are supported by Allen universal stirrups, with knees flexed 90° and thighs both abducted and flexed slightly above horizontal. This position avoids interference with laparoscopic maneuvers and provides some vaginal access. The bladder is continuously drained by a Foley catheter. Sterile preparation and draping are done for abdominal and vaginal access. The VAP is inserted and the seal inflated to preserve pneumoperitoneum while the vaginal cuff is open.

The primary access port placement is done by open or closed technique as indicated at or above the umbilicus, depending upon the size of the uterus. The enlarged uterus tends to interfere with a midline suprapubic port, so in most cases, the author uses two working ports of 10–11 size placed lateral to the inferior epigastric vessels in each lower quadrant of the abdomen. Ports are placed with enough separation to avoid interference. They are positioned with the tips 4 cm inside the peritoneum and then secured in place. High-flow CO_2 insufflation is done through one or two ports as needed, keeping pressure below 15 mm/hg.

The hysterectomy is done by a technique closely following that used in abdominal hysterectomy. The round ligaments are cut and coagulated with ABC. Peritoneum is opened with ABC lateral to the ovarian vessels at the pelvic inlet. Peritoneal incision extends down the anterior broad ligament and across the vesicouterine reflection. Blunt dissection of the bladder is done with the sponge aspirator (Figure 6-4). Dense fibrous adhesions are cut with the harmonic scalpel; loose fibrous bands and small vessels are coagulated with ABC. Adequate

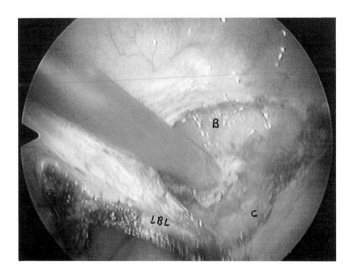

Figure 6-4 Blunt dissection of bladder from cervix with sponge aspirator. B = bladder. C = cervix. LBL = left broad ligament.

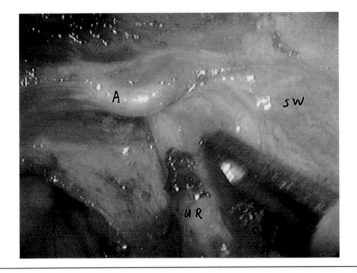

Figure 6-5 Dissection of right ureter and uterine artery. SW = pelvic sidewall. UR = ureter. A = uterine artery. Precise suture ligation of A at this point positively avoids ureteral trauma.

bladder dissection is confirmed by elevation of the vaginal fornices with the end of the VAP.

Retroperitoneal dissection of pelvic sidewalls identifies the course of both ureters and prevents injury of them. The uterus is isolated from the adnexa by placement of a suture ligature around the adnexal bundle and securely tying by extracorporeal technique. This ligature is readily placed through an avascular portion of the posterior broad ligament using a ligature carrier.

If the ovaries are to be removed, the infundibulopelvic vessels are suture ligated. The devascularized adnexae then become cyanotic and may be cut free from the pelvic attachments without significant bleeding (Color plate 4). The adnexae may be cut free from the uterus and deposited in the cul-de-sac, or they may be sutured to the uterine fundus to maximize exposure. If there is ovarian pathology that indicates removal without spillage into the peritoneum, the ovary may be placed within a containment pouch prior to decompression, morcellation, and extraction for pathologic examination.

If the ovaries are to be retained and not impair exposure, the surgeon may choose to leave them attached temporarily and proceed to isolate and suture ligate both uterine arteries. The singly ligated adnexal structures may then be cut free from the devascularized uterus with minimal backbleeding. If exposure is poor, the utero-ovarian attachments may be divided between two ligatures in order to drop the ovaries away from the surgical field.

Exposure of the uterine arteries is facilitated by the assistant, who provides upward countertraction upon one uterine cornu with atraumatic forceps. Blunt dissection of the base of each broad ligament with the sponge aspirator and ABC brings uterine arteries and ureters into full view (Figure 6-5). A laparoscopic hemostat is placed medial to each ureter, to include the uterine artery and part of the cardinal ligament. A suture ligament of #0 Vicryl is then placed and tied securely after the hemostat is removed (Plate 5). Extracorporeal technique is used to tie a firm surgeon's knot backed up by square knots. Pallor and cyanosis of the uterus appear after successful ligation of both uterine arteries and should be observed before either is cut. Troublesome bleeding from major vessels is thus prevented.

If the uterus is bulky, a laparoscope with 30° or 45° angled view is very helpful to visualize the deep pelvic anatomy and facilitate control of the uterine arteries. Once the uterine arteries have been ligated, a laparoscopic scalpel may readily transect them and then amputate the uterine fundus from the cervix. Pelvic exposure is then excellent for completion of the laparoscopic hysterectomy procedure.

If subtotal hysterectomy is planned, the cervical stump is cauterized or sutured for hemostasis and reperitonealized at the surgeon's option. The bulky uterine fundus is stabilized between two laparoscopic tenaculi and morcellated with a laparoscopic scalpel into elongated narrow fragments suitable for extraction through a minilaparotomy incision (Plate 6). After closure of the minilaparotomy, laparoscopic confirmation of hemostasis concludes the procedure.

Total laparoscopic hysterectomy requires that the cervix be cut free from the cardinal, uterosacral, and vaginal attachments. The harmonic scalpel incision of these tissues coagulates most vessels as they are cut, and ABC usually seals larger ones (Figure 6-6). The uterosacral ligaments are suture ligated before incision. The vagina is cut free from the cervix by the harmonic scalpel with minimal bleeding (Plate 7). At the bases of each cardinal ligament, branches of the vaginal arteries are controlled by suture of each lateral vaginal fornix. While the vaginal cuff is open, pneumoperitoneum is retained by the VAP. A laparoscopic tenaculum is passed through the VAP and carefully opened above the colon in view of the laparoscope. The cervix is passed into its grasp by another instrument. As the VAP is removed, the cervix is withdrawn after it through the vagina. Each time the VAP is replaced in the vagina, another fragment of the surgical specimen may be seized with the tenaculum and then extracted for pathologic examination. This process is repeated until all of the specimen has been removed.

If vaginal access is suitable, specimen morcellation may be done

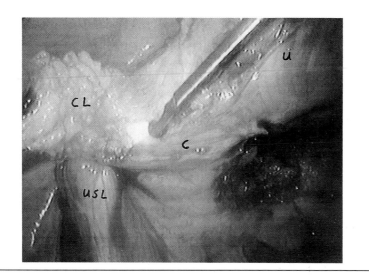

Figure 6-6 Hemostatic dissection of left cardinal ligament from cervix with harmonic scalpel (UltraCision Inc., Smithfield, RI). U = uterus. C = cervix. USL = left uterosacral ligament. CL = left cardinal ligament.

transvaginally, as may the suture repair of the vaginal cuff. The apparent speed and convenience of the vaginal approach is countered somewhat by the time required to reposition the legs, arrange the lights, position the assistant, establish exposure with retractors, and then change gown and gloves before resuming the laparoscopy procedure. In most cases, laparoscopic morcellation is done with better exposure and nearly the same speed as transvaginal. With the VAP in place, the cut edges of vagina are elevated and clearly exposed (Plate 8). Laparoscopic suturing by either interrupted or continuous method requires 10–15 minutes, and results in an accurate, secure, hemostatic vaginal closure. The surgeon may choose laparoscopic or vaginal suturing on a case-by-case basis, as the method expected to be most time-efficient will vary depending upon vaginal anatomy.

Laparoscopic reinspection of the ureters confirms peristalsis and freedom from obstruction. All ligated pedicles are inspected under water. Bleeding points are coagulated or sutured. Access port puncture sites are sutured laparoscopically to prevent hernia formation. Ports are removed in view of the laparoscope to rule out bleeding.

Drains are not routinely used, but when indicated, a 10-mm flat suction drain may be passed through one of the access ports without difficulty and then left in place as the port is removed. The skin is closed around the suction catheter in the usual manner.

Upon completion of the procedure, the vaginal access port is removed and any tissue specimens that may have been stored in it are added to the pathology specimen.

Discussion of surgical technique is incomplete without attention to the management of complications. Preprocedure planning should include assessment of the risk of bleeding or collateral injury of the bowel or urinary tract. Ureteral catheterization or full bowel preparation may be indicated. Furthermore, the procedure should be conducted in a manner that allows efficient response to problems that do occur. Management of hemorrhage is facilitated by the sponge aspirator, which may be used to tamponade vessels with the $1\frac{1}{2}$ inch square sponge it contains, while simultaneously clearing the field by suction through the sponge. Definitive hemostasis is then secured by the appropriate method. If three working ports are necessary to accomplish difficult dissection, placing a fourth port will provide added safety and an extra available grasping instrument should sudden hemorrhage occur. A surgeon qualified to repair an enterotomy, cystotomy, or injured ureter may elect laparoscopic management of such injuries if there is good access and exposure. Laparoscopic repair of injury should only be undertaken when the surgeon is confident of success. Conversion to laparotomy, if indicated, should be early and graceful rather than delayed until the patient is compromised. Fully informed patient consent includes discussion of possible laparotomy.

Clinical results

The author has used the laparoscopic suture method in 170 hysterectomies, of which 117 were laparoscopic hysterectomies, eight were subtotal laparoscopic hysterectomies, and 45 were LAVH. One other case was converted to abdominal hysterectomy because of bleeding and failure to obtain control of uterine arteries by vaginal or laparoscopic approach. Skewing toward laparoscopic hysterectomy was due to the bias introduced by patient referral specifically for laparoscopic hysterectomy, from colleagues who had already selected out candidates for LAVH to be performed by themselves. Operating times ranged from 85 to 270 minutes, with average 150 minutes. Estimated blood loss ranged from 25 to 1200 cc, with average 150 cc. Hospital stay ranged from one to five days, with average 1.2 days. Eight of the last 10 cases were done on an outpatient basis. Two weeks postoperatively, 90% of patients were able to resume customary employment. Six weeks postoperatively, over 95% of patients expressed satisfaction that they had been treated laparoscopically rather than by traditional means.

Patients were treated for a wide variety of conditions typically indicating abdominal hysterectomy. A partial listing includes multiple myomata (500–1500 g) in 11%, severe endometriosis in 18%, adnexal mass in 6%, previous caesarean birth in 9%, severe adhesions due to pelvic inflammatory disease or appendicitis in 4%, familial ovarian cancer syndrome in 3%, and marked obesity in 13%. Adenomyosis in 17% and medically unresponsive menorrhagia in 59% were managed by laparoscopic hysterectomy or LAVH when criteria for vaginal hysterectomy were not fulfilled.

Uterine morcellation was performed in 30% of cases, extensive adhesiolysis in 16%, retropubic urethropexy in 4%, vaginal vault suspension in 3%, appendectomy in 6%, laparoscopic suture of seromuscular bowel injury in 3%, cystotomy repair in 0.6%, and minilaparotomy in 9%.

Complications in the 170 cases were few and not life-threatening. One cystotomy was repaired laparoscopically and healed uneventfully. Five seromuscular bowel injuries were repaired uneventfully by laparoscopic suturing. One trocar injury to an inferior epigastric artery produced increased blood loss, but was controlled by laparoscopic suture. Five patients experienced increased blood loss due to severe endometriosis-induced fibrosis of the cul-de-sac and vaginal cuff. One required transfusion. One patient experienced increased blood loss during partial vaginectomy for VIN 3/CIN 3, which was done prior to the laparoscopic procedure. Two patients experienced postoperative ileus, which resolved fully without sequelae. One patient was readmitted for treatment of pelvic infection, which promptly resolved after parenteral antibiotic therapy. One small bowel obstruction occurred due to herniation into a right lower quadrant trocar puncture site. It did not require bowel resection and cleared completely upon release from the abdominal wall. The author now routinely sutures the port puncture sites laparoscopically to prevent herniation.

Conclusion

Laparoscopic suturing and knot tying are advanced skills that add flexibility and extend the therapeutic range of operative laparoscopy into the realm of reparative surgery. The technical challenges for the surgeon are amply rewarded by the enhanced recovery of patients who are thereby enabled to avoid laparotomy. It should be emphasized that laparoscopic hysterectomy does not compete with or replace vaginal hysterectomy. Vaginal hysterectomy is expected to remain an important technique and will continue to be advisable in 25 to 30% of all cases. LAVH may allow an additional 25 to 30% of patients to avoid laparotomy, but the available vaginal exposure remains a constraint upon its general application.

The suture method makes laparoscopic hysterectomy a viable alternative to abdominal hysterectomy, and may so serve for an additional 25 to 30% of patients. There will probably be an irreducible 10 to 20% of patients who will continue to require abdominal hysterectomy for treatment of their illness. Clearly, this revolution in the hysterectomy procedure will require some time, as it requires the retraining of thousands of surgeons. In the author's opinion, mastery of operative laparoscopy by the suture method is essential to achieve maximum conversion of hysterectomy to minimally invasive surgery.

Suggested reading

1 Meilahn JE. The need for improving laparoscopic suturing and knot-tying. J Laparoendoscopic Surg 1992;2(5):267.

2 Pietrafitta JF. A technique of laparoscopic knot tying. J Laparoendoscopic Surg 1992;2(5):273–275.

3 Sharpe LA. A new device and method for extracorporeal knot tying in laparoscopic surgery. J Gynecol Surg 1994;10:27–31.

4 Kennedy JS. A technique for extracorporeal suturing. J Laparoendoscopic Surg 1992;2(5):269–272.

5 Kadar N, Reich H, Liu CY, Manko GF, Gimpelson R. Incisional hernias after major laparoscopic gynecological procedures. Am J Obstet Gynecol 1993;168(5):1493–1495.

6 Carlson KJ, Nichols DH, Schiff I. Indications for hysterectomy. New Engl J Med 1993;328(12):856–860.

7 Friedman A, Haas ST. Should uterine size be an indication for surgical intervention in women with myomas? Am J Obstet Gynecol 1993;168(3, part 1):751–755.

8 Reich H, DeCaprio J, McGlynn F. Laparoscopic hysterectomy. J Gynecol Surg 1989;5(2):213–216.

9 Padial JG, Sotolongo J, Casey MJ, Johnson C, Osborne NG. Laparoscopy-assisted vaginal hysterectomy: report of seventy-five consecutive cases. J Gynecol Surg 1992;8(2):81–85.

10 Woodland MB. Ureter injury during laparoscopy-assisted vaginal hysterectomy with the endoscopic linear stapler. Am J Obstet Gynecol 1992;167(3):756–757.

11 Liu CY. Laparoscopic hysterectomy. J Reprod Med 1992;37(4):351–354.

12 Summit RL, Stovall TG, Lipscomb GH, Ling FW. Randomized comparison of laparoscopy-assisted vaginal hysterectomy with standard vaginal hysterectomy in an outpatient setting. Obstet Gynecol 1992;80(6):895–901.

13 Nezhat F, Nezhat C, Gordon S, Wilkins E. Laparoscopic versus abdominal hysterectomy. J Reprod Med 1992;37(3):247–250.

14 Canis M, Mage G, Wattiez A, Pouly JL, Chapron C, Bruhat MA. Vaginally assisted laparoscopic radical hysterectomy. J Gynecol Surg 1992;8(2):103–105.

15 Goodman MP, Johns DA, Levine RL, Reich H, Levinson CJ, Murphy AA, et al. Report of the study group: advanced operative laparoscopy (pelviscopy). J Gynecol Surg 1989;5(4):353–360.

16 Howard FM. Breaking new ground or just digging a hole? An evaluation of gynecologic operative laparoscopy. J Gynecol Surg 1992;8(3):143–158.

17 Grody MHT. Vaginal hysterectomy: the large uterus. J Gynecol Surg 1989;5(3):301–312.

18 Nezhat C, Nezhat F, Nezhat C. Operative laparoscopy (minimally invasive surgery): state of the art. J Gynecol Surg 1992;8(3):111–141.

19 Semm K, Friedrich ER. Operative manual for endoscopic abdominal surgery. Chicago: Year Book Medical Publishers, 1987.

20 Soderstrom RM. Operative laparoscopy. The masters' techniques. In: Sands LE, ed., Principles and techniques in gynecologic surgery. New York: Raven Press, 1993.

7 Subtotal Hysterectomy

THOMAS LYONS

History and rationale for subtotal hysterectomy

Why subtotal hysterectomy?

There is ample data in the world literature that document the significantly decreased morbidity of subtotal versus total hysterectomy. In a world-wide review, Tervilä calculated that the mortality associated with subtotal hysterectomy was 0.71%, as opposed to 1.03% in total hysterectomy (1). Nevertheless, most gynecologists continue to perform total hysterectomy rather than supravaginal amputation because total hysterectomy generally is thought to reduce patients' risk of cervical carcinoma.

Taken from large population European studies with meticulous long-term follow-up, data published during the 1980s suggests the risk of carcinoma of the cervical stump following subtotal hysterectomy has been overestimated. The evidence indicates rather that supravaginal amputation, or supracervical hysterectomy, may not be associated with a higher occurrence of morbidity due to cervical carcinoma. Reporting on a series of more than 2,700 cases completed between 1952 and 1978, Kilkku et al. (2) cited an incidence of carcinoma of the cervical stump of 0.11%—significantly lower than the incidence of 0.56% reported in prior series of hysterectomies. Two important factors may account for this difference. First, the advent of routine Pap smears in the U.S. around 1958 has made noninvasive cytologic surveillance a commonplace tool for gynecologists. Second, in the Finnish series reported by Kilkku (3), all cases involved perioperative electrocoagulation of the ectocervix, specifically as prophylaxis against carcinoma of the cervix. In most reported series of supracervical subtotal hysterectomy, the incidence of carcinoma in the existing cervical stump is lower (.1% to 1.4%) than in a similar population with intact uteri (.4% to 5%).

These re-examinations of previous assumptions have led to a resurgence of interest in subtotal hysterectomy, which has been well documented as the lower morbidity abdominal hysterectomy procedure (4). This interest has combined with more broad-based experience among surgical gynecologists with laparoscopy, leading to the advent of a new procedure, laparoscopic supracervical hysterectomy (LSH), which can be a considerably easier procedure for most practitioners than the technically difficult laparoscopically assisted vaginal hysterectomy (LAVH).

[84]

There are several alternatives to LAVH currently in practice. One is the classic method for laparoscopic subtotal hysterectomy assisted by SEMM (serrated macro morcellator) that includes coring of the uterine cervix from below, but this classic abdominal SEMM hysterectomy (CASH) procedure has specific limitations: it is not appropriate for larger uteri; it requires special equipment (the SEMM Morcellator); and it may be associated with significant postoperative bleeding problems. Another is the procedure developed by Pelosi that uses a single umbilical puncture. This technique is difficult, however, and, in many cases, not applicable.

LSH is, in essence, a reprise of the oldest hysterectomy technique using the newest laparoscopic methods, which results in a product that is highly satisfactory to the patient. It must be said that every hysterectomy patient is not a candidate for LSH; however, in light of the Thompson data in TeLinde (4) that establishes lower morbidity, it becomes difficult to find appropriate indications for removal of the cervix, with the clear exception of invasive carcinoma of the cervix or carcinoma of the endometrium. Barring the relatively infrequent diagnoses of carcinoma, subtotal hysterectomy may be appropriate. This procedure should be discussed with the patient as an option, particularly because the new data does not support the rationale for total hysterectomy as necessary prophylaxis for carcinoma of the cervix (4).

Morbidity of subtotal hysterectomy versus total hysterectomy

Recent re-examinations of mortality trends have begun to dispel the widely held notion that supracervical hysterectomy is associated with a higher level of cervical carcinoma. This author's own experience has demonstrated statistically significant differences in the comparative morbidity of LAVH and LSH.

The author has reported on a recent series of 100 patients who underwent surgical procedures (Table 7-1) (5). Fifty patients had LAVH and 50 patients underwent LSH using the same energy sources and surgical methods. There was a statistically significant decrease in the morbidity of the LSH cases in five categories: operative time, estimated blood loss (EBL), hospital stay, return to work, and return to normal activity (Figure 7-1).

The average operative time for LAVH was 27 minutes longer (18.6%) than for LSH. Calculated blood loss was much higher in LAVH due almost exclusively to a 175-cc average loss at the vaginal site. The author found several other morbidity parameters were increased in the LAVH group as well, including vaginal discharge, postoperative bladder symptomology (frequency, spasm, urgency), postoperative bowel symptomology, and increased back pain. Decreased postoperative libido and decreased coital frequency were also noted in the LAVH group. Neither group had significant complications, which is especially remarkable in light of the large average size (> 75 kg) of the patients in this study.

Data published throughout the 1980s support these findings (2). They also suggest that abdominal subtotal hysterectomy may offer con-

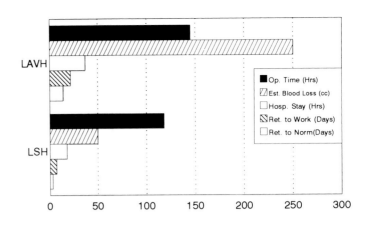

Figure 7-1 In a series of 100 patients (50 LAVH, 50 LSH) with similar demographic characteristics, significantly lower morbidity was associated with LSH than LAVH in terms of operative time, estimated blood loss, length of hospital stay, return to work, and return to normal activity.

Table 7-1 Comparative statistics of LAVH versus LSH

Patient demographics	LAVH	LSH
Average age	43	42
(years)	(30–81)	(28–72)
Weight (kg)	80.1	85.9
Height (cm)	146	155
Prior abdominal surgery	2.1	1.6
(average number of procedures)		

siderable benefits in terms of reduced morbidity, especially with regard to urinary and sexual function posthysterectomy.

In a study of postoperative symptoms of hysterectomy, Kilkku examined 212 patients who had undergone hysterectomy with regard to urinary symptoms (specifically, pollakisuria, nocturia, and dysuria) (6). Prior to hysterectomy, more than one fourth of the abdominal hysterectomy patients (27.6%) and nearly half (48.6%) of the supracervical hysterectomy patients (supravaginal amputation) experienced pollakisuria. Nocturia and dysuria were present in about 10% of patients in both groups.

Postoperatively, nocturia and dysuria disappeared more frequently in patients undergoing supracervical hysterectomy than in abdominal hysterectomy cases. Twelve months postoperatively, there was a statistically significant difference in complaints of pollakisuria—10.3% of supracervical hysterectomy patients and 13.5% of abdominal hysterectomy patients.

In a later study of subjective bladder symptoms and incontinence (7), Kilkku noted a dramatic decrease in the sensation of residual urine after micturition in abdominal supracervical hysterectomy patients as compared to total abdominal hysterectomy (TAH) patients (10.3% and 22.1% respectively at one year postoperatively). A highly statistically significant decrease also was noted for incontinence: at one year postoperatively, 22.6% of supracervical hysterectomy patients reported incontinence (versus 47.7% preoperatively), while 28.8% of abdominal hysterectomy patients experienced incontinence (as compared to 36.2% preoperatively).

Based on this extensive series, Kilkku concludes that the reduced

[86]

morbidity in urinary symptoms seen with supracervical amputation may result from the less extensive manipulation of the bladder during this procedure. While he further suggests that support provided by the retained cervical stump and the uterosacral ligaments also may help reduce urinary symptoms, these studies clearly suggest that the greater reduction in urinary symptoms seen in the supracervical hysterectomy group is primarily due to the type of procedure performed rather than to other factors.

Kilkku conducted a similar series of follow-up studies of hysterectomy patients' postoperative symptoms specifically concerning effects on sexual function (8). He concluded that total abdominal hysterectomy was associated with a highly significant decrease in frequency of orgasms. Abdominal supracervical hysterectomy, however, was not associated with decreased orgasmic frequency. Dyspareunia was relieved by both abdominal hysterectomy and supracervical hysterectomy, but more so by the supracervical procedure. As with his studies of urinary function, Kilkku concludes that the greater radicality of TAH has a greater effect on orgasmic frequency than does supracervical hysterectomy. It is felt by the present author and others (9) that the maintenance of an intact Frankenhäuser's plexus and its neurologic contribution may explain this phenomenon. Another factor that was not charted but could be important is the length of abstinence associated with surgery.

Although sexual function is understood to be a complex reaction to many interrelated factors, studies clearly suggest that leaving a patient's cervix intact may be less disruptive to sexual function. These data, combined with data from studies on postoperative urinary and bowel symptomology, present a convincing case for supracervical hysterectomy in patients where there is no medically compelling reason for cervical removal.

Data showing reduced postoperative morbidity with LSH are convincing. Nevertheless, the fact remains that the morbidity associated with either this procedure or LAVH is small, compared to TAH. Where large statistical differences do exist becomes quite apparent once economic morbidity is factored in (Figure 7-2). In light of growing eco-

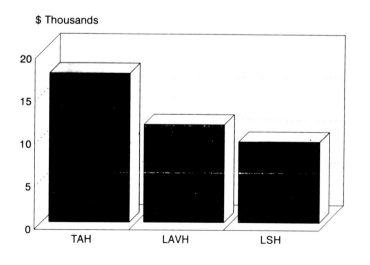

Figure 7-2 Comparative economic morbidity of total abdominal hysterectomy (TAH), laparoscopically assisted vaginal hysterectomy (LAVH), and laparoscopic supracervical hysterectomy (LSH). Average cost per procedure ($ thousands).

[87]

nomic sensitivity to health-care costs, a procedure such as LSH that offers reduced hospital stay, more rapid return to work, and more rapid return to normal activity emerges as a desirable alternative.

Laparoscopic supracervical hysterectomy

Every hysterectomy patient is not a candidate for laparoscopic hysterectomy. However, the indications for LSH are much the same as those for LAVH. These include:
• dysfunctional bleeding (excluding patients who are candidates for endometrial ablation or total vaginal hysterectomy)
• pelvic or abdominal pain
• adnexal masses with indications for hysterectomy
• endometriosis requiring definitive surgery (patients should not have extensive cervical disease that would require removal of the cervix)
• known or suspected adhesive disease, or pelvic inflammatory disease
• indicated appendectomy with hysterectomy indications
• difficult vaginal hysterectomy requiring removal of the adnexa (i.e., in a nulligravida or a patient with vaginal or anatomical abnormalities)
• tubo-ovarian abscess
Contraindictions for this procedure are endometrial cancer and invasive cervical cancer.

Patient preparation

In preparation for the procedure, full patient consent for laparotomy should be obtained, as with all operative laparoscopic procedures. The patient also should be encouraged to participate in a full discussion of the supracervical approach, and this discussion should be documented in the patient's chart. The discussion—and the documentation—should emphasize the need for continued cytologic surveillance.

All attendant laparoscopic technologies should be available, including a contact Nd:YAG laser system, bipolar Kleppinger forceps, Endoloops, ligatures, ligaclips, and endocutters.

Techniques for laparoscopic supracervical hysterectomy

Laparoscopic supracervical hysterectomy (Lyons technique)

The OR setup for LSH is shown in Figure 7-3. A double-monitor setup is used, with the primary surgeon on the patient's left, the scrub nurse at the patient's foot, and the secondary or assistant surgeon on the patient's right. A bipolar cautery unit is basic equipment for this procedure.

Use of a cutting instrument that coagulates as it cuts is imperative to the success of this procedure, which requires frequent desiccation and division of highly vascularized tissues. Both the ultrasonically activated scalpel (harmonic scalpel) and Nd:YAG laser scalpel have been used with significant success in LSH. Monopolar/cold scissors also have been used in the technique described.

The patient is positioned for exploratory laparotomy in the modified dorsal lithotomy position with Allen stirrups. A Cohn cannula is placed as a uterine manipulator with a single-toothed tenaculum.

Trocars are placed as noted in Figure 7-4. A Hasson or open cannula is placed at the subumbilical site. A secondary 10/11-mm trocar is placed in the midline, approximately three to four fingerbreadths above the symphysis pubis. Additional secondary 5-mm trocars are placed bilaterally, well lateral to the rectus muscle, approximately four finger breadths above the symphysis pubis.

Because of the risk of bladder or bowel damage during trocar placement, placement of the Hasson cannula using an open technique is strongly recommended. In a review of penetration injuries associated with placement of a Veress needle and/or a sharp trocar, Perone (10) noted that 14% of unintended laparotomies associated with laparoscopic tubal sterilization resulted from difficulty in entering the peritoneal cavity. Use of the open technique significantly decreases risk of penetration injuries and facilitates trocar placement in patients with prior abdominal surgeries and large patients and also facilitates removal of the specimen at the end of the case.

The open technique for placing a Hasson cannula requires an initial 2-cm linear subumbilical incision. To facilitate entry into the abdominal cavity, dissection of this incision is carried toward the umbilical aponeurosis. This dissection is important, especially in large patients. Once the open cannula is positioned, it is sutured into place using two 0-Vicryl sutures.

The operative laparoscope is introduced and an initial exploration of the abdomen is performed. This exploration includes any pathology as well as a careful evaluation of the anatomy for placement of the secon-

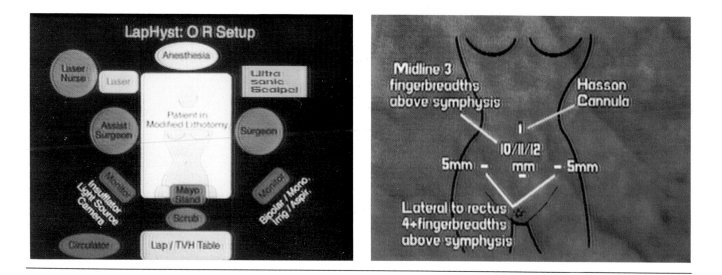

Figure 7-3 OR setup—laparoscopic supracervical hysterectomy.   **Figure 7-4** Trocar placement—LSH.

dary trocars. The type of trocars used depends on the patient's size and on the attendant pathology.

The surgeon may vary placement of the secondary trocars based on a variety of factors, including the patient's size, the presence of adhesive disease, or the presence of attendant pathology. All secondary trocars should be placed under transillumination and direct visualization with the laparoscope. Placement of secondary trocars in a somewhat higher position than that noted in traditional laparoscopic descriptions may aid the surgeon in moving and manipulating the uterus while performing hysterectomy.

After the first secondary trocar is placed, it may be necessary to manipulate and move the bowel before inserting the other trocars. The lateral trocars are placed lateral to the rectus muscles, well lateral to the epigastric vasculature.

Exploratory laparoscopy

Following placement of all secondary trocars, exploratory laparoscopy is performed. A thorough exploration of pelvic and abdominal contents allows the surgeon to clearly identify the pelvic structures in addition to any attendant pathologies outside the pelvis (Figure 7-5).

Adhesiolysis/initial dissection

If the ovaries are to be left in place, dissection usually begins on the right side. Adhesiolysis is performed to take down adhesions along the lateral pelvic wall. After careful visualization of the ureter, the infun-

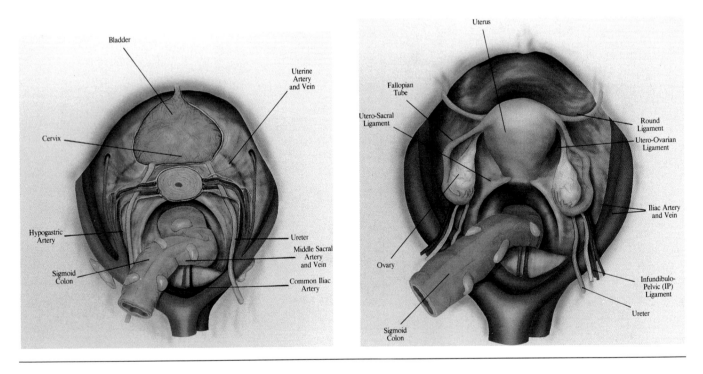

Figure 7-5A Female pelvis (cut-away uterine vessel level).

Figure 7-5B Female pelvis (posterior cul-de-sac view).

dibulopelvic ligaments are desiccated with bipolar cautery and divided using the Nd:YAG laser scalpel. It may not be necessary to fully dissect out the ureter if it is readily visualized. The ureter usually can be visualized well below the ligamentous structure (Figures 7-6). If uterolysis is indicated, the lateral pelvic sidewall is opened above the ligament, and isolation of the IP ligament and ureter is accomplished in the traditional fashion.

On the left side, in order to visualize the area of the ureter, it often is necessary to take down the congenital adhesions of the sigmoid colon (Figure 7-7).

Once the area of the ureter has been opened and the left ureter is identified, desiccation of the right infundibulopelvic ligament is accomplished with bipolar Kleppinger forceps. Multiple desiccations may be necessary to thoroughly coagulate this ligament. The ligament is then divided with a laser, ultrasonically activated scalpel, or scissors, and a 0-PDS Endoloop is used to secure this vascular structure (Plate 9).

The remainder of the broad ligament tissues are divided using a cutting tool. An instrument that both cuts and coagulates facilitates this dissection by coagulating the small capillary bleeders found in these tissues. For the cutting tool to work to its best advantage, it usually is necessary to place countertraction, or "organize" the tissue.

If the ovary is to be left in place, the round ligament and uterovarian pedicle are lifted, visualized well away from associated structures, and desiccated with the bipolar cautery unit (Figure 7-8). Because of the vascularity associated with the tissues lateral to the uterus, multiple desiccations may be required. Thorough desiccation of these structures decreases back-bleeding.

Once the round ligament is fully desiccated, a laparoscopic scalpel or

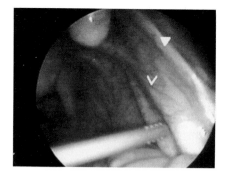

Figure 7-6 Desiccation of the infundibulopelvic ligament. After clearly visualizing the ureter, the infundibulopelvic ligament is desiccated using the Kleppinger bipolar forceps. Here, the ureter is visualized well below the infundibulopelvic ligament.

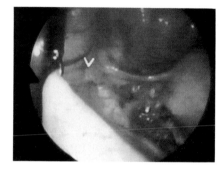

Figure 7-7 Adhesiolysis—congenital adhesions of the sigmoid colon.

Figure 7-8 Desiccation and division of the round ligament and utero-ovarian pedicle.

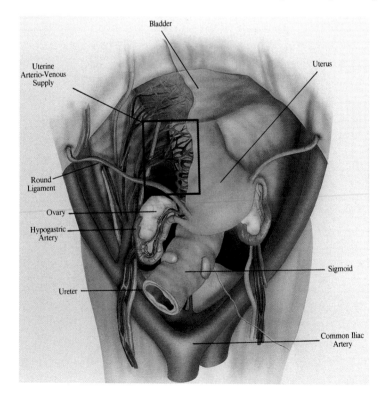

Bladder

Uterine Arterio-Venous Supply

Uterus

Round Ligament

Ovary

Hypogastric Artery

Sigmoid

Ureter

Common Iliac Artery

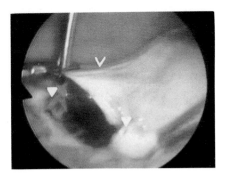

Figure 7-9 Bladder flap dissection.

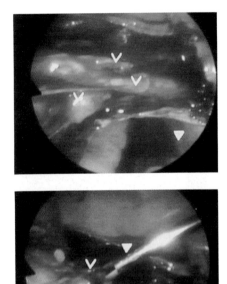

Figures 7-10A and 7-10B Skeletonization of the uterine vessels. Dessication of uterine vessels.

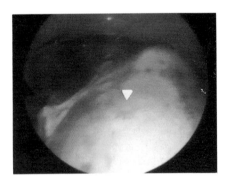

Figure 7-11 Desiccation of the uterine vessels.

scissors are used to divide the ligament. Any areas of bleeding encountered during division are desiccated again using the bipolar cautery unit. During this process, periodic reidentification of the ureter is suggested since anatomic landmarks appear somewhat different with laparoscopic procedures.

Division of the round ligaments allows opening of the uterovesical fold of the peritoneum for dissection of the bladder flap (Figure 7-9, Plate 10). Laparoscopy allows excellent visualization in this area. In patients who have had prior cesarean section, scarring of the bladder flap may make opening of the uterovesical fold of peritoneum more difficult. Several techniques may be employed to accomplish this dissection, including aquadissection, endoscopic Kittner, or sharp dissection. Careful attention to detail on the bladder flap dissection opens the uterine fossa and allows visualization of the uterine vasculature.

Dissection should be carried across from the left lateral side to the midline and the midline condensation ligament. This is divided using the scalpel. The posterior leaf of the broad ligament must then be addressed.

Dissection of the posterior leaf of the broad ligament allows the ureter to splay laterally, well away from the dissection process (Plate 11), and allows skeletonization of the uterine vessels. The uterine vasculature is then dissected and skeletonized, using both blunt and sharp dissection.

Once the uterine vessels can be skeletonized—just as in an abdominal case—they can be coagulated with bipolar forceps, well away from the ureter. Multiple desiccations are necessary as the uterine vessels are quite tortuous, and multiple arcades can be viewed throughout the area lateral to the uterus (Figures 7-10A and 7-10B).

Both uterine vessels should be carefully desiccated prior to attempting division of either vascular pedicle. Without bilateral desiccation, significant back-bleeding can occur during opening of the uterine vessels. The surgeon can easily tell when the vessels have been completely desiccated, as the uterus, when visualized, rapidly will appear cyanotic (Figure 7-11).

After the uterine vessels have been completely desiccated, the vessels are divided.

With bilateral division of the uterine vessels completed, the remainder of the uterine amputation is accomplished, coring down into the cervix, beginning at or below the level of the internal os, in a reverse conization fashion (Figure 7-12).

The division of the lower uterine segment begins with division of the endocervical canal. Using a laser or ultrasonically activated scalpel, the cut is made down into the endocervical canal using the uterine manipulator that has been placed in the canal as a marker for its location. Once the canal is reached, dissection proceeds to the lateral and posterior aspects of the uterus (Figure 7-13). The Cohn cannula is removed and the remainder of the uterus is amputated.

Once the uterus has been amputated, the endocervical canal is coagulated using the laser, with monopolar or bipolar cautery. Any remaining endocervical tissue higher in the canal is desiccated or vaporized (Figure

7-14). The surgeon should note a good conization or coring effect of the cervix.

The anterior and posterior leaves of peritoneum are plicated over the cervical stump using a 2-0 Vicryl suture in a mattress fashion. Use of extracorporeal knotting techniques will greatly expedite this process. The surgeon also may use an endoscopic stapler in this area to close the peritoneal surface over the cervical stump (Figures 7-15A and 7-15B).

The abdomen is cleaned of any collected blood, fluids, or other products and inspected for any signs of bleeding, while decreasing intra-abdominal pressure to 8 mm/Hg or less. Any areas of bleeding should be attended to carefully using the bipolar forceps, the harmonic ball, or the Nd:YAG hemostasis tip.

Appendectomy or other procedures may be performed as necessary prior to removal of the uterus. A posterior culdoplasty is performed routinely, using a 2-0 Vicryl suture in a purse-string fashion, which plicates the uterosacral ligaments posteriorly. Again, use of extracorporeal knotting speeds the procedure. A modified Moskowitz posterior culdoplasty is accomplished readily and definitely occludes the posterior cul-de-sac, giving the vaginal vault excellent support.

Only after thorough hemostasis has been assured is the uterus bifurcated or morcellated using sharp dissection. Uterine tissue is then removed through the anterior abdominal wall subumbilical site (Figure 7-16). This site is easily extended slightly to accomodate the larger uterine fundus or leiomyoma. During this process, the operative laparoscope is moved to the lower 10/11-mm trocar for direct visualization of removal of the uterus, which is teased out through the open cannula site.

The trocars are then removed under direct visualization, as they were placed. Larger incisional sites are closed in layers. The 5-mm trocar sites are closed with steristrips unless bleeding is evident.

The patient is allowed to recover with a Foley catheter in place for four to six hours. Early ambulation is encouraged, and discharge usually can be accomplished within 18 hours. The patient may resume normal activity as soon as she feels comfortable doing so.

Classic abdominal SEMM hysterectomy (SEMM technique)

The CASH procedure takes advantage of the sophisticated apparatus and instrumentation now available in a novel technique of intrafascial hysterectomy without colpotomy. This technique satisfies cancer prophylaxis and leaves the pelvic floor topography intact.

The patient is placed in a modified lithotomy position using Allen stirrups. A Foley catheter is in place, and, after sounding the uterus, an appropriate manipulator is inserted.

Four trocars are positioned in a "Z" fashion: first, a 5-mm trocar is inserted through either the right or left rectus muscle; after thorough inspection of the abdominal and pelvic cavities, this trocar is replaced with a 10-mm optic trocar. Two 5-mm trocars are placed suprapubically, under direct vision, lateral to the deep epigastric vessels. An additional 10-mm trocar is placed suprapubically.

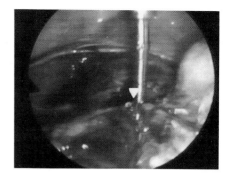

Figure 7-12 Beginning amputation of the uterus.

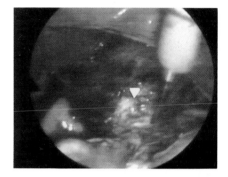

Figure 7-13 Division of the lower uterine segment and endocervical canal.

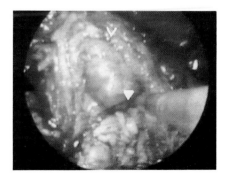

Figure 7-14 Endocervical electrocoagulation.

[93]

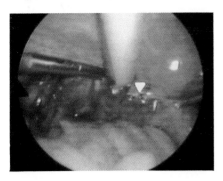

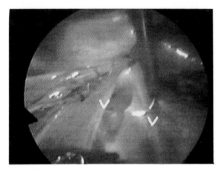

Figure 7-15A and 7-15B Plication of the posterior peritoneum over the cervical stump.

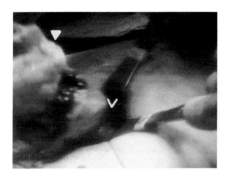

Figure 7-16 Removal of the uterus.

The patient is reclined in a 15° Trendelenburg position, which displaces the bowel out of the pelvis.

The CASH procedure begins with injection of the round ligament and the anterior and posterior leaves of the broad ligament with dilute Pitressin solution to facilitate aquadissection. The ligaments are coagulated and divided with a hook scissors. This creates a large window in the bloodless space of the broad ligament. Pedicles are secured with 0-PDS and/or 0-catgut Endoloops.

A 0-Vicryl ligature is placed through the window in the broad ligament to ligate either the infundibulopelvic ligament or the utero-ovarian ligament, depending on whether or not adnexae are to be removed. A second ligature is placed on the uterine side. The ligament is divided between the two ligatures using a hook scissors, electrocautery, or a laser.

The anterior and posterior leaves of the broad ligament are then infiltrated with Pitressin. The bladder flap is developed and the posterior leaf is dissected down to the uterosacral ligament, as in laparotomy. Vessels are exposed carefully with a Kittner dissector; this dissection exposes ascending branches of the uterine artery and displaces the ureter laterally. No further dissection of the bladder, cardinal, or uterosacral ligaments is necessary.

A 0-PDS Endoloop is then placed over the uterus so it loosely hugs the isthmus of the cervix at the level of the insertion of the uterosacral ligament.

The next stage of the CASH procedure is performed vaginally. The uterine manipulator is removed and the cervix is grasped with a single-tooth tenaculum at 12 and six o'clock. The cervix is infiltrated with Pitressin until blanched. The cervix is dilated to Hegar 5, and a Schiller test is performed to be sure the complete squamocolumnar junction is included in the morcellator.

The uterus is perforated with a rod, ensuring that the cervix and corpus uteri form a straight cylinder. This facilitates complete removal of Müllerian tissue.

The tissue cylinder is cored out using a calibrated uterine resection tool (CURT) set. The appropriate size CURT set (10 mm to 20 mm) is determined by sonography and/or manual examination. The tissue cylinder is gently removed along with the whole CURT set. The prepared PDS Endoloop is immediately applied to occlude the cervical canal and both ascending branches of the uterine artery. A small piece of Surgicel™ is placed into the cervical canal and a loose 4 × 4 sponge is placed into the vagina (the sponge is removed at the end of the procedure).

The final steps of the CASH procedure are accomplished abdominally. Two more 0-PDS Endoloops are placed around the cervix. The corpus uteri is amputated with a hook scissors and "parked" in the right pelvic gutter until the end of the procedure. An additional 0-catgut Endoloop is placed over the cervical stump for security. A point coagulator is used to coagulate the surface of the cervical stump as well as the pedicles of the round ligament and the infundibulopelvic or utero-ovarian ligaments.

[94]

The 10-mm trocar site is dilated to 15 or 20 mm and a SEMM set is inserted for removal of the surgical specimen. One or two o-Vicryl sutures peritonealize the pelvic floor.

After thorough irrigation with lactated Ringer's solution, trocars are removed under direct vision. The 10-mm trocar sites are closed with staples, and the smaller wounds are closed with steristrips.

The CASH procedure avoids removal of the cervix, which is the more difficult, bloody, and risky part of abdominal hysterectomy. However, by eliminating the entire mucosa, including the squamocolumnar junction, it also reduces the possibility of neoplasia. CASH thus reduces the risk of cervical stump carcinoma and also the need for extensive dissection of the bladder. By preserving the cardinal ligament support (with its blood and nerve supply) and the cervicovaginal unit, CASH preserves pelvic support and thus minimizes effects on sexual function.

Single-puncture supracervical hysterectomy

Recently, Pelosi reported on four patients who underwent single-puncture supracervical hysterectomy and bilateral salpingo-oophorectomy for benign uterine disease, with highly satisfactory outcomes (11).

Following placement of an intrauterine cannula for uterine manipulation, a 10-mm operative laparoscope is inserted transumbilically. Standard operative laparoscopic instruments, including unipolar and bipolar electrosurgery instruments, scissors, a blunt probe, and aquadissection devices, are introduced through the 5-mm operative channel of the laparoscope.

The surgical steps of the single-puncture supracervical hysterectomy, as described by Pelosi, are performed much as those used in a traditional abdominal hysterectomy. The uterovarian ligament and associated structures are desiccated and then transected. To facilitate separation of the bladder from the uterus, the bladder is partially distended with methylene blue. Aquadissection and sharp dissection are used to identify the ureters and to skeletonize the uterine vessels, which are then coagulated and transected. To facilitate amputation of the cervix below the internal cervical os, the upper half of the cardinal ligaments are coagulated and transected. A conization-like technique, similar to the one described by Lyons, is used to amputate the cervix.

Prior to removal, the uterus is bisected symmetrically. Extension of the umbilical incision is accomplished by severing the peritoneum and the fascial layer with a scissors introduced through the operative channel of the laparoscope. This step results in sudden loss of pneumoperitoneum, which is restored by clamping the edges of the extended incision with an Allis clamp to produce a seal around the cannula.

Using grasping forceps, one-half of the bisected uterus is grasped and brought up to the umbilicus. The Allis clamp is released and the operative laparoscope, its cannula, and the grasping forceps holding the specimen are removed from the abdominal cavity as a single unit. Kocher clamps are used to facilitate removal of the specimen.

Pelosi reported no intraoperative complications and uncomplicated postoperative recovery in all four cases. Patients were discharged within 72 hours and resumed normal daily activities and work within 14 days. In the discussion of these cases, Pelosi notes that, in addition to offering a miminally invasive procedure, the single umbilical puncture approach offers the advantages of lower cost, simplicity, avoidance of complications associated with multiple punctures, and superior cosmetic results.

Issues in subtotal hysterectomy

Despite the gradual resurgence of subtotal hysterectomy, total hysterectomy remains the method of choice among surgeons today. The primary criticism of subtotal hysterectomy revolves around the risk of cervical cancer in patients with a retained cervical stump—a criticism that has been laid to rest, once and for all, by Tervilä (1) and others. More recently, the Human Papilloma Virus (HPV) epidemic has added further fuel to the argument favoring total hysterectomy, with the view that the high incidence of HPV-related and other cervical dysplasias continues to justify total hysterectomy.

The fact remains that epidemiologic evidence simply does not support radical removal of the cervix as the solution to eliminating cervical cancer risk. In the U.S., the number of hysterectomies per year peaked at one million in 1975, 17 years after the start of routine Pap smears as part of standard gynecologic practice. Since cytologic surveillance became routine, there has been a four-fold decrease in deaths from cervical cancer and a corresponding decline in the number of hysterectomies (Figure 7-17). There also has been rapid advancement in alternative, less invasive treatments for cervical disease, which has played an important role in managing the morbidity associated with the rise in HPV-related and other cervical dysplasias. The net sum of all of these factors is that there is no reason to continue to assume that total hysterectomy is the best choice for all patients.

Figure 7-17 Cervical cancer and cervical dysplasia versus incidence of hysterectomy. Epidemiologic evidence does not support the belief that total hysterectomy effectively reduces risk of cervical cancer.

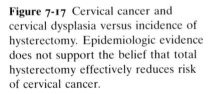

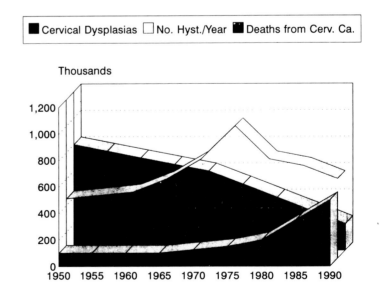

Today, in an era when the gynecologist is able to evaluate and treat cervical disease with multiple less invasive local therapies, including Pap smear, colposcopy and biopsy via directed biopsy, cold knife conization, laser therapy and electrosurgical excisional therapy, supracervical hysterectomy is an appropriate therapeutic alternative. The growing list of widely available local therapies for cervical disease make it difficult to find indications for removal of the cervix beyond that of invasive carcinoma of the cervix or carcinoma of the endometrium.

Much in the same way as laparoscopic cholecystectomy has been adopted rapidly by the surgical community, laparoscopic hysterectomy is an enticing new procedure for the surgical gynecologist. However, the laparoscopic techniques required to perform laparoscopic hysterectomy are extensive and must be performed only after adequate training and education in operative laparoscopy.

LSH is a considerably easier approach for the trained gynecologic surgeon as it does not add a difficult vaginal procedure to the termination of an already difficult laparoscopic procedure. The relatively easier nature of the procedure should decrease bladder and ureteral injuries, and it should be appropriate for more cases, including large leiomyomata or Müllerian abnormalities. Finally, LSH provides better stability for the pelvic floor, allowing further supportive procedures to be accomplished more readily. The modified Moskowitz procedure has become a routine portion of the Lyons procedure, and anterior (round ligament) suspensions have been accomplished with success in vault prolapse patients. In addition, the ability to successfully use uterosacral colpopexy may be significantly improved by using the cervical stump as an anchor for these suspension procedures.

All of these factors contribute to this author's belief that, in the U.S., LSH will allow a greater number of abdominal hysterectomy patients to be converted to the laparoscopic approach, producing a significant effect on morbidity, mortality, and cost. It is also conceivable that vaginal hysterectomy can be addressed supracervically and further increase utilization of this procedure. Patient acceptance of these procedures is at least as impressive as the morbidity and mortality statistics.

References

1 Tervilä L. Carcinoma of the cervical stump. Acta Obstet Gynecol Scand 1963; 42:200–210.

2 Kilkku P, Grönroos M. Peroperative electrocoagulation of endocervical mucosa and later carcinoma of the cervical stump. Acta Obstet Gynecol Scand 1982;61: 265–267.

3 Kilkku P, Grönroos M, Rauramo L. Supravaginal uterine amputation with peroperative electrocoagulation of endocervical mucosa. Description of method. Acta Obstet Gynecol Scand 1985;64:175–177.

4 Thompson JD. Hysterectomy. In: Thompson JD, Rock JA, eds. TeLinde's operative gynecology, 7th ed. Philadelphia: JB Lippincott, 1992:686–687.

5 Lyons TL. Laparoscopic supracervical hysterectomy: a comparison of morbidity/ mortality results with LAVH. J Reprod Med 1993;38(7):763–767.

6 Kilkku P, Hirvonen T, Grönroos M. Supravaginal uterine amputation vs. abdominal

hysterectomy: the effects on urinary symptoms with special reference to pollakisuria, nocturia and dysuria. Maturitas 1981;3:197–204.

7 Kilkku P. Supravaginal uterine amputation versus hysterectomy with reference to subjective bladder symptoms and incontinence. Acta Obstet Gynecol Scand 1985; 64:375–379.

8 Kilkku P, Grönroos M, Hirvonen T, Rauramo L. Supravaginal uterine amputation vs. hysterectomy: effects on libido and orgasm. Acta Obstet Gynecol Scand 1983; 62:147–152.

9 Hasson HM. Cervical removal at Hysterectomy for benign disease: risks and benefits. J Reprod Med 1993;38(10):781–791.

10 Perone N. Laparoscopy using a simplified open technique: a review of 585 cases. J Reprod Med 1992;37(11):921–924.

11 Pelosi MA, Pelosi MA III. Laparoscopic supracervical hysterectomy using a single-umbilical puncture (mini-laparoscopy). J Reprod Med 1992;37(9):777–784.

8 The Traditional Approach to Uterine Malignancies

LAURA WILLIAMS

Cancer of the uterine corpus is the most common gynecologic malignancy, accounting for almost as many new cases per year as cancer of the ovary and cervix combined (1) (Figure 8-1). In 1992, approximately 32,000 women were diagnosed with uterine cancer and 4000 patients died of the disease, making corpus cancer the seventh leading cause of cancer death in women. Over three-quarters of patients are diagnosed in the postmenopausal period, and fewer than 5% are under the age of 40 (2). Risk factors for the disease include hypertension, diabetes, and obesity; thus, uterine cancer remains a formidable problem in an aging and potentially medically compromised population.

NEXT PARA RESET

Unlike ovarian carcinoma, endometrial cancer, the most common uterine malignancy, presents as a Stage I tumor in over 75% of cases (1). This century has seen a myriad of treatment strategies utilizing radiation, surgery, and hormone therapy for the treatment of the disease confined to the uterus by clinical assessment. With the improvement of anesthetic techniques and postoperative care, the role of the primary surgical approach has assumed greater importance. Sentinel surgical-pathologic staging studies performed by the Gynecologic Oncology Group (GOG) (3,4) in the 1980s have helped define prognostic factors for lymph node metastasis, extrauterine spread, and recurrence in patients who appear preoperatively to have disease confined to the uterus. These studies provide the basis for individualization of postoperative radiation therapy to the pelvis and are the foundation for further clinical investigation into the role of adjuvant treatment. In 1988, the International Federation of Gynecology and Obstetrics (FIGO) adopted a surgical staging schema that

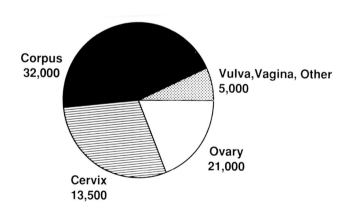

Figure 8-1 Estimated incidence of gynecologic malignancies in 1992.

[99]

mandated primary removal of the pelvic organs and lymph nodes to accurately stage corpus cancer (5). In this chapter, we will review the rationale and technique of the hysterectomy in the contemporary surgical approach to cancer of the uterine corpus and its precursor lesions.

Endometrial hyperplasia

Precursor lesions to cancer of the endometrium have been categorized according to architectural and cytologic atypia and analyzed with respect to carcinogenic potential. In a 1985 report (6), Kurman and associates described the long-term follow-up of 170 patients with endometrial hyperplasia. *Simple hyperplasia* was defined as a mild to moderate overgrowth of crowded endometrial glands with irregular borders; this category included lesions formerly referred to as cystic or adenomatous hyperplasia. *Complex hyperplasia* was characterized by marked structural abnormalities and back-to-back crowding, but no significant cytologic abnormality was present. *Atypical hyperplasia* contained glands with varying degrees of nuclear atypia and loss of polarity. When followed for propensity to progress to invasive adenocarcinoma of the endometrium, the investigators found that fewer than 2% of patients with hyperplasias without cytologic atypia progressed to carcinoma, no matter how architecturally complex, whereas 23% of patients with cytologic atypia (atypical hyperplasia) progressed to cancer (Table 8-1). The International Society of Gynecologic Pathologists recognized the importance of the presence of cytologic atypia in the current classification of endometrial hyperplasia (Table 8-2).

The management of patients with endometrial hyperplasia takes into account the age and reproductive desires of the patient as well as the patient's medical condition and the histologic features of the lesion. Individualization of treatment based on these factors supports the role of hysterectomy in the management of some patients. Table 8-3 illustrates a treatment scheme. Because of the low risk of progression to carcinoma, patients without cytologic atypia are often successfully managed with progestational agents, and ovulation induction may be attempted in women who desire fertility. Some have advocated dilatation and curettage of the uterus as an adjunct to medical treatment (7). Numerous progestational agents and methods of administration have achieved favorable outcomes (7–9).

Table 8-1 Long-term follow-up of patients with endometrial hyperplasia

Type of hyperplasia	Number	Progressed to cancer	%
Simple	93	1	1
Complex	29	1	3
Simple atypical	13	1	8
Complex atypical	35	10	29

Reprinted from Kurman R, Kaminski P, Norris H. The behavior of endometrial hyperplasia: a long-term study of untreated hyperplasia in 170 patients. Cancer 1985;56:403–412.

Table 8-2 Classification of endometrial hyperplasia.

Simple hyperplasia
Complex hyperplasia (adenomatous hyperplasia without atypia)
Atypical hyperplasia (adenomatous hyperplasia with atypia)

For patients with atypical cytologic changes, in whom the risk of progression to invasive cancer is substantially increased, hysterectomy is considered appropriate initial treatment in the operative candidate. Kurman and Norris (10) analyzed the hysterectomy specimens of 28 women under the age of 35 who had atypical hyperplasia in uterine scrapings on previous dilatation and curettage and found that 11% of uteri contained well-differentiated, noninvasive adenocarcinoma of the endometrium. In contrast, approximately 60% of women over the age of 55 had residual carcinoma in the specimen (7). For this reason, many authors support transvaginal or transabdominal hysterectomy for the initial treatment in operative candidates and reserve hormonal therapies for patients who are poor operative risks. The surgical approach in patients with presumed atypical endometrial hyperplasia should take into account the considerable liklihood of finding adenocarcinoma in the final hysterectomy specimens.

Endometrial cancer

Historical perspective

In his 1882 book, Dr. T. S. Wells describes what he believes to be the first gravid hysterectomy performed in England (11). This procedure was performed in 1881 in a 37-year-old woman at approximately 25 weeks' gestation who suffered chronic vaginal discharge from epithelioma of the cervix extending into the uterine cavity. Dr. Wells' assistant records the times and events of the procedure:

Table 8-3 Management of endometrial hyperplasia

	Desires fertility	Does not desire fertility and operable	Postmenopausal or inoperable
Simple hyperplasia	Ovulation induction Progestational agents	Progestational agents	Progestational agents
Complex hyperplasia	Ovulation induction Progestational agents	Progestational agents	Progestational agents
Atypical hyperplasia	Ovulation induction High-dose progestins	Hysterectomy	High-dose progestins

2.35 P.M.   Patient began to inhale methylene.

2.41   "   Catheter and plugging vagina.

2.50   "   Incision in abdominal wall.

2.53   "   Uterus drawn out.

2.56   "   Sutures in upper part of abdominal wall, dividing broad ligaments and vagina, removing foetus and securing vessels, till

3.10   "   Uterus removed.

3.40   "   Ligature of vessels and sutures of vagina and broad ligaments.

3.50   "   Closing of wound and dressing.

3.55   "   Patient in bed.

Her postoperative course was complicated by fascial dehiscence, purulent vaginal discharge and a burn to the lower extremity from a hot water bottle, but she returned to her home in Kent, satisfactorily recovered, one month later. This case served to reignite Wells' interest in the hysterectomy for the treatment of cancer of the womb as attempts to extirpate the uterus by Blundell and others early in the 19th century had met with dismal results. However, with a reported 75% mortality rate and considerable difficulty managing ureters at abdominal exploration, and despite therapeutic success reported by Dr. W.A. Freund in 1878 (12), in the late 19th century, Wells and other surgeons came to favor vaginal hysterectomy for the treatment of uterine cancer (11).

Subsequent to these surgical reports, the Curies reported the discovery of radium in 1886 (13), and the following decades saw the incorporation of radiation therapy techniques into the management of carcinoma of the uterine corpus. In 1916, Howard Kelly reported the use of radium in a substantial number of endometrial cancer patients, and 13 years later, Healy and Brown (14) described the integration of surgery and radiation techniques for the treatment of the disease. In the 1930s, Heyman described a technique of packing the uterus with radium capsules (15) prior to a planned hysterectomy. This technique underwent modifications by others, but by the 1940s, the standard approach to carcinoma of the endometrium had become preoperative radiation therapy followed by total abdominal hysterectomy (TAH) and bilateral salpingo-oophorectomy (BSO) (15). In the 1950s, the radical hysterectomy and pelvic lymphadenectomy was popularized in the United States by Meigs and Brunschwig, but due to the elderly and often medically compromised nature of endometrial cancer patients, this operation proved to be inappropriate for the majority of cases, and cure rates were not significantly better than for simple hysterectomy and radiation alone (15). In this decade, Swedish investigators reported improved cure rates when radiation was delivered to the vaginal vault after hysterectomy, and this practice has continued to the present day without the benefit of a randomized prospective assessment of efficacy (16). Therefore, in the decades prior to the introduction of the surgical staging schema by FIGO, the initial treatment approach to primary adenocarcinoma of the endometrium was not standardized, consisting of intracavitary or external radiation therapy, preceded or followed by hysterectomy, often without assessment of intra-abdominal or nodal metastases.

Contemporary surgical management

FIGO STAGING FOR CARCINOMA OF THE CORPUS: In 1977, the Gynecologic Oncology Group undertook a prospective surgical pathologic staging study in order to evaluate the prognostic factors for extrauterine spread or relapse in patients who appeared preoperatively to have cancer confined to the uterine corpus (3,4). Six-hundred and twenty-one clinical stage I endometrial cancer patients underwent TAH, BSO, selective pelvic and para-aortic lymphadenectomy, and pelvic washings. Five uterine and five extrauterine risk factors were identified as predictors of lymph node metastasis or recurrence (Table 8-4). Of these risk factors, histologic cell type and tumor grade may be determined prior to surgery, but the remaining risk factors are assessed only after histologic evaluation of the specimen. This prospective evaluation led FIGO to adopt a primary surgical approach to corpus cancer, incorporating many of these prognostic factors into the staging schema (17) (Table 8-5). There remains, however, considerable controversy among gynecologic oncologists regarding the role of retroperitoneal lymph node sampling in patients with tumors that have limited myometrial invasion, and this will be discussed below.

SURGICAL TECHNIQUE: An adequate surgical incision is necessary to perform the hysterectomy, explore the upper abdomen, and, if appropriate, to accomplish pelvic and para-aortic lymph node sampling. Often, this is a vertical incision that can be extended around the umbilicus; however, in some morbidly obese patients, a wide upper abdominal transverse incision may be necessary. Pelvic washings are obtained upon opening the abdomen and entering the pelvis, and lymph-node-bearing areas of the retroperitoneum and pelvic structures are then examined for gross metastases. BSO and TAH with a vaginal cuff are performed as the sentinel procedures. The cardinal ligaments are clamped outside the pubocervical fascia, and the vesicouterine ligament (roof of the ureter) and para-

Table 8-4 Risk factors in endometrial carcinoma

Uterine factors	Extrauterine factors
Histologic type	Adnexal metastasis
Grade	Intraperitoneal spread
Myometrial invasion	Positive peritoneal cytology
Isthmus-cervix extension	Pelvic node metastasis
Vascular space invasion	Para-aortic node metastasis

Reprinted with permission from Park R, Grigsby P, Muss H, Norris H. Corpus: epithelial tumors. In: Principles and practice of gynecologic oncology. Philadelphia: JB Lippincott, 1993:663–693.

Table 8-5 FIGO staging for carcinoma of the corpus uteri

Stage IA G123	Tumor limited to endometrium
Stage IB G123	Invasion to less than one-half the myometrium
Stage IC G123	Invasion to more than one-half the myometrium
Stage IIA G123	Endocervical glandular involvement only
Stage IIB G123	Cervical stromal invasion
Stage IIIA G123	Tumor invades serosa and/or adnexa, and/or positive peritoneal cytology
Stage IIIB G123	Vaginal metastasis
Stage IIIC G123	Metastasis to pelvic and para-aortic lymph nodes
Stage IVA G123	Tumor invasion of bladder and/or bowel mucosa
Stage IVB	Distant metastases including intra-abdominal and/or inguinal lymph nodes

Histopathology—degree of differentiation:

Cases of carcinoma of the corpus should be classified (or graded) according to the degree of histologic differentiation, as follows:

G1 = 5% or less of a nonsquamous or nonmorular solid growth pattern
G2 = 6–50% of a nonsquamous or nonmorular solid growth pattern
G3 = more than 50% of a nonsquamous or nonmorular solid growth pattern

Notes on pathologic grading:

(1) Notable nuclear atypia, inappropriate for the architectural grade, raises the grade of a grade 1 or grade 2 tumor by 1.
(2) In serous adenocarcinomas, clear-cell adenocarcinomas, and squamous cell carcinomas, nuclear grading takes precedence.
(3) Adenocarcinomas with squamous differentiation are graded according to the nuclear grade of the glandular component.

Rules related to staging:

(1) Because corpus cancer is now staged surgically, procedures previously used for determination of stages are no longer applicable, such as the findings from fractional D&C to differentiate between stage I and stage II.
(2) It is appreciated that there may be a small number of patients with corpus cancer who will be treated primarily with radiation therapy. If that is the case, the clinical staging adopted by FIGO in 1971 would still apply, but designation of that staging system would be noted.
(3) Ideally, width of the myometrium should be measured along with the width of tumor invasion.

metrial tissue are left intact (Figure 8-2). The uterus is then examined for depth of myometrial invasion, and in many centers, a frozen section is performed to establish the FIGO grade of the tumor (Figure 8-3).

LYMPH NODE SAMPLING: If retroperitoneal lymph nodes are to be sampled based on the intraoperative assessment of tumor grade and myometrial invasion, systematic removal of these nodes is then accomplished. The sentinel pelvic nodal groups to be removed include the common iliac, external iliac, and obturator lymph nodes (3). To accomplish lymph node sampling, an incision is made in the peritoneum over the common iliac artery and extended down the external iliac artery to the circumflex iliac vein. The lymphatics and nodal tissue surrounding these vessels and

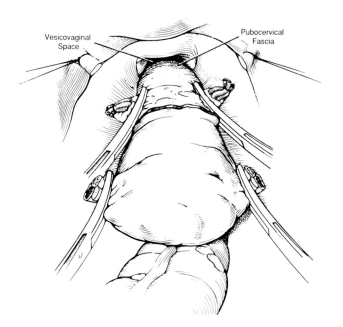

Figure 8-2 Extrafascial hysterectomy for adenocarcinoma of the endometrium.

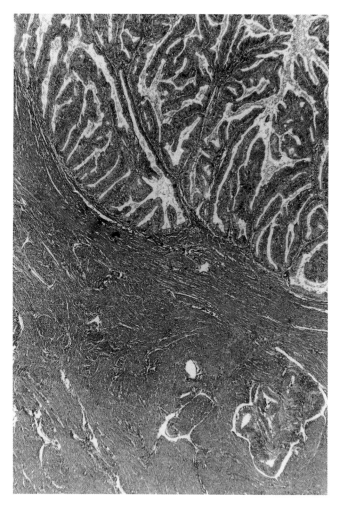

Figure 8-3 Well-differentiated (FIGO grade 1) adenocarcinoma of the endometrium.

beneath the external iliac vein above the obturator nerve are excised. To remove the para-aortic nodes, the peritoneal incision over the common iliac artery is extended superiorly and the precaval fat pad from the aortic bifurcation is removed superiorly. If necessary, the left and right colon may be mobilized medially to gain exposure to these areas.

Most gynecologic oncologists agree that lymph node sampling is not necessary in patients with tumor limited to the endometrium, as fewer than 1% of these patients have metastases to retroperitoneal nodes, regardless of tumor grade. Based on the prospective surgical-pathologic data generated by the GOG (3), Park and associates (18) recommend that pelvic and para-aortic lymph node sampling be performed for the following reasons: myometrial invasion greater than 50%, extension of tumor to the cervix or lower uterine segment, extrauterine metastasis detected at laparotomy, the presence of serous, clear-cell, squamous or undifferentiated cell types, or clinically enlarged lymph nodes (Table 8-6) The authors point out that patients with grade 2 or 3 lesions and inner one-half myometrial invasion as the only risk factor have less than 5% chance of nodal metastases, and in these patients, node sampling may not be warranted (18). Because the overall surgical complication rate

Table 8-6 Indications for retroperitoneal node sampling

Myometrial invasion $> 1/2$
Isthmus-cervix extension
Extrauterine spread
Serous, clear, squamous, or undifferentiated cell types
Enlarged lymph nodes

Reprinted with permission from Grigsby C, Perez C, Camel H. Stage II carcinoma of the endometrium: results of therapy and prognostic factors. Int J. Rad Oncol Bio Phys 1985.

for node sampling in this group of patients is 20% (3), we recommend individualized assessment of the surgical approach in patients with intermediate risk factors. For patients with myometrial invasion greater than 50%, node sampling is recommended, particularly if adjuvant therapy will be directed by the findings.

STAGE 2 ENDOMETRIAL CANCER: Primary surgical staging is employed for the medically operable patient who has occult spread to the cervix. Prior to the surgical staging schema proposed by FIGO, patients believed to have extension of endometrial tumor to the cervix (clinical stage 2) often underwent radiation followed by surgery as the initial approach to treatment. Although no randomized prospective trial has validated this approach, commonly employed treatment plans included whole pelvic external radiation followed by intracavitary cesium and simple hysterectomy. In small retrospective series, survival for this group of patients ranges from 70-85% (19–21). This approach or intracavitary radiation followed by simple hysterectomy 48 hours later (22) are treatment methods often still employed for the patient with gross cervix involvement. Medically inoperable patients are treated by radiation therapy alone; in these patients, survival drops to approximately 50%. Radical hysterectomy and bilateral pelvic lymphadenectomy, historically employed for some patients with cervix involvement, does not appear to offer improved survival compared with radiation and simple hysterectomy, and morbidity is substantially higher (24).

Tumors of the uterine stroma

According to SEER (Surveillance, epidemiology, and end results) estimates, the incidence of sarcomas of the uterus ranges from one to 2.3 cases per 100,000 (23). Overall, these tumors account for less than 5% of all cancers of the corpus (18). The most common histologic subtypes in order of decreasing incidence are mixed Müllerian tumor (carcinosarcoma) followed by leiomyosarcoma and endometrial stromal sarcoma. Carcinosarcoma peaks in incidence between the ages of 65 and 74, although leiomyosarcoma is typically found in younger women (23). In some series of carcinosarcomas, a history of pelvic radiation can be obtained in up to 30% of cases and may precede the development of the uterine tumor by two to 20 years (24,25). Carcinosarcomas, high grade leiomyosarcomas, and endometrial stromal sarcomas are characterized by early lymphatic dissemination and hematogenous spread, whereas low grade leiomyosarcomas and stromal sarcomas are more likely to remain confined to the uterus and to be cured by surgery. When these low grade neoplasms do recur, they are often amenable to surgical debulking, providing the patient with a long disease-free interval.

The surgical approach

The standard initial surgical approach to the patient with uterine carcinosarcoma consists of extrafascial TAH and BSO. The benefits of extended surgical staging have not been verified in a prospective fashion, but in patients found to have extrauterine metastases, aggressive surgical intervention or complete surgical staging is unlikely to alter the outcome (26). In patients with disease confined to the uterus or cervix (stage 1 or 2), the five-year disease-free survival is approximately 50%. In some retrospective series, adjunctive radiation therapy has improved locoregional control, but does not appear to significantly alter survival (23). Some patients with disease confined to the corpus may be candidates for adjuvant chemotherapy protocols designed to decrease relapse risk; the Gynecologic Oncology Group is currently studying ifosfamide and cisplatin in this clinical setting.

Retroperitoneal lymph node sampling is rarely useful in patients with leiomyosarcoma of the uterus, as the majority of patients with the nodal metastases have clinically enlarged nodes (27). TAH and BSO are indicated for patients who have a high grade leiomyosarcoma or for patients with low or intermediate grade tumors who are not interested in future fertility. For the patient who has undergone myomectomy to find a high grade sarcoma involving a myoma (> 10 mitoses per 10 high power fields), hysterectomy is recommended as the majority of these patients will relapse if no further surgery is performed (28). If a low or intermediate grade lesion is found to involve a fibroid tumor (5–9 mitoses per 10 high power fields without significant nuclear atypia), the patient may need no further treatment. O'Connor and Norris reported that 13 of 14 patients with cellular leiomyomata treated by myomectomy alone had favorable outcomes (29).

In a 1990 publication from Memorial Sloan-Kettering Cancer Center (30), the recurrence risk for patients who underwent hysterectomy for low grade endometrial stromal sarcoma without oophorectomy was 100% versus 43% for patients who had TAH with BSO performed. These tumors are known to contain high levels of estrogen and progesterone receptors and are hormonally sensitive. In some cases, surgery more extensive than TAH is necessary to completely remove the pelvic tumor, and this assessment is often made at the time of surgery (18).

Gestational trophoblastic disease

The implementation of effective chemotherapy has limited the role of hysterectomy in the treatment of gestational trophoblastic disease (GTD).

For patients with nonmetastatic GTD, primary remission rates range from 77–98% with single-agent chemotherapy, and overall cure rates approach 100% in most series (31). Prior to the identification of methotrexate as an active agent, Brewer and colleagues reported a 40% two-year survival in patients treated by hysterectomy alone (32). Nevertheless, there still appears to be a role for hysterectomy in the patient undergoing chemotherapy. Hammond and associates, from Duke University (33), reported the treatment results of patients with nonmetastatic and low-risk metastatic disease. In the patients who underwent hysterectomy during the first cycle of chemotherapy (Figures 8.4 and 8.5), the number of cycles needed to produce remission was reduced and the total duration of therapy was shortened. Hysterectomy is, therefore, recommended early in the course of chemotherapy treatment for the patient with nonmetastatic or low-risk metastatic disease who does not wish to retain fertility. These same investigators (33) did not observe the same benefit to early hysterectomy in patients with high-risk metastatic GTD. In these patients, hysterectomy may be reserved as a salvage treatment for the occasional patient who has persistent disease confined to the uterus (31).

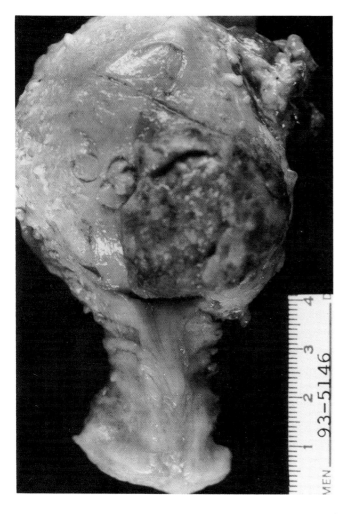

Figure 8-4 Hysterectomy specimen with persistent choriocarcinoma following chemotherapy.

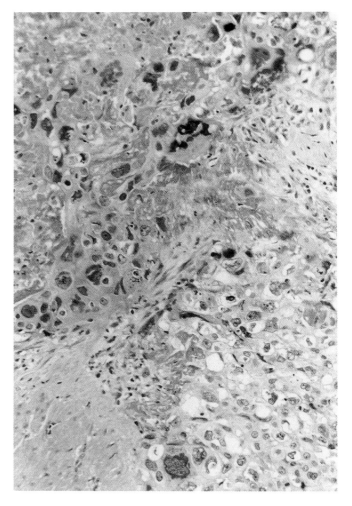

Figure 8-5 Photomicrograph of choriocarcinoma demonstrating malignant cytotrophoblasts and syncytiotrophoblasts.

References

1 Boring C. Cancer statistics, 1992. Ca Cancer J Clinicians 1992;42:19–38.

2 Gallup D, Stock R. Adenocarcinoma of the endometrium in women 40 years of age or younger. Obstet Gynecol 1984;64:417.

3 Creasman W, Morrow C, Bundy B, et al. Surgical pathologic spread patterns of endometrial cancer—a GOG study. Cancer 1987;60:2035–2041.

4 Morrow C, Bundy B, Kurman R, et al. Relationship between surgical-pathologic risk factors and outcome in clinical stage I and II carcinoma of the endometrium. Gynecol Oncol 1991;40:55–65.

5 FIGO. Corpus cancer staging. Int J Obstet Gynecol 1989;28:190.

6 Kurman R, Kaminski P, Norris H. The behavior of endometrial hyperplasia: a long-term study of untreated hyperplasia in 170 patients. Cancer 1985;56:403–412.

7 Richart R, Ferenczy A, Gelfand M, Kurman R. Conservative or aggressive management of early Ca? Contemp Obstet Gynecol 1984;253–273.

8 Ferenczy A, Gelfand M. Hyperplasia vs. neoplasia: two tracks for the endometrium? Contemp Obstet Gynecol 1986;79–96.

9 Trope C, Lindahl B. Premalignant features of the endometrium: clinical features and management. In: Gynecologic oncology. Edinburgh:Churchill Livingston, 1992:747–751.

10 Kurman R, Norris H. Evaluation of criteria distinguishing atypical endometrial hyperplasia from well-differentiated carcinoma. Cancer 1982;49:2547–2549.

11 Wells TS. On partial amputation and on complete excision of the uterus. In: On ovarian and uterine tumors: their diagnosis and management. London: J and A Churchhill, 1882:518–530.

12 Freund W. A new method for extirpation of the whole uterus. Berl Klin Wochenschr 1878:275–417.

13 Curie P, Curie MP, Bemont G. Sur une nouvelle substance fortement radioactive contenue dans la pechblende (not presented by M. Becherel). Compt Rend Acad Sci (Paris) 1888;1215.

14 Healy W, Brown R. Experience with surgical and radiation therapy in carcinoma of the corpus uteri. Am J Obstet Gynecol 1939;38:1–13.

15 Nori D. Principles of radiation therapy in the management of carcinoma of the endometrium. In: Radiation therapy of gynecological cancer. New York: Alan R. Liss, 1987:115–146.

16 Kottmeier H. The place of radiation therapy and of surgery in the treatment of uterine cancer. J Obstet Gynaecol Br Emp 1955;62:737–746.

17 International Federation of Gynecology and Obstetrics. Annual report of the results of treatment in gynecologic cancer. Int J Gynecol Obstet 1989;28:189–190.

18 Park R, Grigsby P, Muss H, Norris H. Corpus: Epithelial tumors. In: Hoskins WJ, Perez CA, Young RC, eds. Principles and practice of gynecologic oncology. Philadelphia: JB Lippincott, 1993:663–693.

19 Grigsby PW, Perez CA, Camel HM, Kao MS, Galakatos AE. Stage II carcinoma of the endometrium: results of therapy and prognostic factors. Int J Rad Oncol Biol Phys 1985;11(1):1915–1923.

20 Greven K, Olds W. Radiotherapy in the management of endometrial carcinoma with cervical involvement. Cancer 1987;60:1737–1740.

21 Landgren R, Fletcher G, Delclos L, Wharton, JT. Irradiation of endometrial cancer in patients with medical contraindications to surgery or with unresectable lesions. Am J Roentgenol Rad Ther Nuc Med 1976;126:148–154.

22 Trimble E, Jones IH. Management of stage II endometrial adenocarcinoma. Obstet Gynecol 1988;71:323–326.

23 Hannigan E, Curtin J, Silverberg S, Thigpen J, Spanos W. Corpus: mesenchymal tumors. In: Hoskins WJ, Perez CA, Young RC, eds. Principles and practice of gynecologic oncology. Philadelphia: JB Lippincott, 1993:695–714.

24 Dinh T, Slavin RE, Bhagavan B, Hannigan EV, Jamson EM, Yodell RB. Mixed müllerian tumors of the uterus: a clinicopathologic study. Obstet Gynecol 1989;74:388–392.

25 Doss L, Lorens A, Hernandez E. Carcinosarcoma of the uterus: a 40-year experience from the state of Missouri. Gynecol Oncol 1984;18:43–53.

26 Podczaski E, Woomert C, Stevens C Jr. Management of mixed mesodermal tumors of the uterus. Gynecol Oncol 1989;32:240–244.

27 Leibsohn S, d'Ablaing G, Mishell D, Schlaerth J. Leiomyosarcoma in a series of hysterectomies performed for presumed uterine sarcomas. Am J Obstet Gynecol 1990;162:968–974.

28 Berchuck A, Rubin S, Hoskins W, et al. Treatment of uterine leiomyosarcoma. Obstet Gynecol 1988;71:845–850.

29 O'Connor D, Norris H. Mitotically active leiomyomas of the uterus. Hum Pathol 1990;21:223–227.

30 Berchuck A, Rubin S, Hoskins W, et al. Treatment of endometrial stromal tumors. Gynecol Oncol 1990;36:60–65.

31 Soper J, Hammond C, Lewis J. Gestational trophoblastic disease. In: Hoskins WJ, Perez CA, Young RC, eds. Principles and practice of gynecologic oncology. Philadelphia: JB Lippincott, 1993:795–825.

32 Brewer J, Smith R, Pratt G. Absolute survival rates of 122 patients treated by hysterectomy. Am J Obstet Gynecol 1963;841–845.

33 Hammond C, Weed J, Currie J. The role of operation in the current therapy of gestational trophoblastic disease. Am J Obstet Gynecol 1980;136:844–858.

9 Laparoscopic Approaches to the Care of Uterine Cervical Cancer

GUY J. PHOTOPULOS

Cervical cancer occurs in 13,000 women annually in the United States, causing 4,500 deaths (1). Treatment for invasive and advanced cancer requires extensive, complex surgery or radiation. In addition to the cases of invasive cervical cancer, 600,000 preinvasive lesions occur annually but are usually managed with hysterectomy or, more frequently, by a lesser procedure. Many people, encouraged by recent advances in operative laparoscopy, have applied these laparoscopic techniques to the management of cervical cancer; we will review these techniques and indicate how they are being used to benefit cervical cancer care.

Uterine cervical cancer

Treatment of invasive cervical cancer is determined primarily by tumor stage (Table 9-1) (2), depth of invasion, and volume. Preinvasive cancer is usually treated locally by cone biopsy, loop excision, laser, or cryotherapy and uterine preservation. Microinvasive squamous cell carcinoma not exceeding 3-mm invasion without vascular space involvement usually requires simple hysterectomy. However, a modified radical hysterectomy provides better treatment for lesions just exceeding these limits (IA2) (3). Stages IB and IIA lesions less than 4 cm in diameter receive either radical hysterectomy and pelvic lymphadenectomy or radiation (4), while radiation with or without a standard hysterectomy (5,6,7) serves better for large, "barrel" cancers confined to the cervix. Radiation is the primary treatment of cancer extending beyond the cervix and the adjacent vagina (stages IIB, III, and IVA); however, surgical staging has served in planning the dose and distribution of the radiation (8,9,10,11). Therefore, surgery is used either to remove the cervical cancer or to define more accurately the extent of tumor and provide direction for optimal radiation therapy.

Laparoscopic procedures suited to the care of cervical cancer

Diagnostic laparoscopy

First, we will discuss laparoscopic procedures with potential use in the care of cervical cancer, and then we will review their application to specific clinical situations arising in cervical cancer. Diagnostic laparoscopy,

Table 9-1 Staging of carcinoma of the uterine cervix

AJC primary	FIGO tumor (T)	
TX		Primary tumor cannot be assessed
TO		No evidence of primary tumor
Tis	O	Carcinoma in situ
T1	I	Cervical carcinoma confined to uterus (extension to corpus should be disregarded)
T1a	Ia	Preclinical invasive carcinoma, diagnosed by microscopy only
T1a1	Ia1	Minimal microscopic stromal invasion
T1a2	Ia2	Tumor with invasive component 5 mm or less in depth taken from the base of the epithelium and 7 mm or less in horizontal spread
T1b	Ib	Tumor larger than T1a2
T2	II	Cervical carcinoma invades beyond uterus but not to pelvic wall or to the lower third of vagina
T2a	IIa	Without parametrial invasion
T2b	IIb	With parametrial invasion
T3	III	Cervical carcinoma extends to the pelvic wall and/or involves lower third of vagina or causes hydronephrosis or nonfunctioning kidney
T3a	IIIa	Tumor involves lower third of the vagina, no extension to pelvic wall
T3b	IIIb	Tumor extends to pelvic wall or causes hydronephrosis or nonfunctioning kidney
T4*	IVa	Tumor invades mucosa of bladder or rectum and/or extends beyond true pelvis

Regional lymph nodes (N)

Regional lymph nodes include paracervical, parametrial, hypogastric (obturator), common, internal and external iliac, presacral and sacral.

NX	Regional lymph nodes cannot be assessed
NO	No regional lymph nodes metastasis
N1	Regional lymph nodes metastasis

Distant metastasis (M)

MX	Presence of distant metastasis cannot be assessed
MO	No distant metastasis
M1	IVb distant metastasis

*Presence of bullous edema is not sufficient evidence to classify a tumor T4.
Beahrs OH, Henson DE, Hutter RVP, Myers MH, eds. Manual for Staging of Cancer, 3rd ed. Philadelphia: JB Lippincott, 1988, 151–153.

the easiest laparoscopic procedure, provides excellent inspection of the peritoneum for metastatic cancer by using a 5- or 10-mm laparoscope, usually placed at the umbilicus; the entire abdomen and pelvis are inspected methodically just as at open laparotomy. Through a 5-mm trocar, the pelvis and upper abdomen are lavaged with saline for cytology. Adhesions are carefully cut to permit safe, thorough inspection. Small metastases appear as white, slightly raised nodules most frequently found on the uterosacral ligaments, adnexa, or pelvic peritoneum. Image magnification through the scope and video monitor reveals lesions not even seen at routine, surgical inspection. Biopsies of peritoneum should be easily ob-

[112]

tained by grasping the peritoneum adjacent to a suspicious lesion or simply at a random site using dissecting forceps through a 5-mm trocar placed 3–5 cm superior and medial to the anterior-superior iliac spine (on the left for a right-handed surgeon). Scissors placed through a second 5-mm trocar 3–5 cm superior and to the left (again, for a right-handed surgeon) of the umbilical laparoscope are used to incise and then dissect under the peritoneum. Before cutting the peritoneum, however, care must be taken to identify major vessels and the ureters. Also, coagulation should not be used until the specimen has been removed to avoid histological, thermal artifact. In order to help with insertion and biopsy, a third 5-mm operative port may be placed 3–5 cm medial and superior to the right anterior-superior iliac spine; it is not always necessary but is needed, for example, during para-aortic node biopsies and more advanced operative procedures.

During inspection of the pelvis, common, internal, and external iliac vessels are identified and visually traced. Any irregular elevations of the peritoneum caused by an enlarged node suspicious of cancer should be looked for at this time. A suspicious node should be removed by cutting the overlying peritoneum and lifting the node gently from the neighboring vessel. Care should be taken, as the soft wall of a vein may be elevated with the node; lack of depth perception through the scope deserves special mention here, as it could be very easy to cut the vessel. However, by pushing with closed scissors *toward* the vessel, the node will separate from the vessel wall so that a free space between the two is seen. Usually a node has small vascular attachments proximally and distally that are cut with low-power coagulation. Alternatively, a large fixed node that cannot be removed safely should be aspirated under direct vision with a needle, or a shave biopsy from the node's surface is adequate.

Pelvic lymphadenectomy

Pelvic lymphadenectomy, a much more difficult procedure than inspection and biopsy, begins with incision of the peritoneum lateral and parallel to the hypogastric arteries. They are easily seen extending in looping manner from posterior-lateral at the common iliac artery bifurcation to anterior-medial. With the artery held in a medial direction, the scissors are used to push the fat and nodes laterally away from the artery and toward the obturator nerve (Figure 9-1)—cutting is usually not required, particularly near the nerve and not until it has been identified. Obturator nodes are then removed with blunt dissection (Figure 9-2). Nodes over the external iliac artery and vein are next removed. Usually these vessels are separated from the lateral psoas muscle and from each other to allow for removal of all external iliac nodes. The dissection may be extended to include nodes of the distal common iliac artery; care must be taken not to damage the ureter as it crosses the bifurcation of the common iliac artery. Also, a troublesome artery and vein run laterally from the proximal, external iliacs to the psoas muscle. The accessory obturator vein deserves special note; when present, it enters the distal-posterior, external iliac

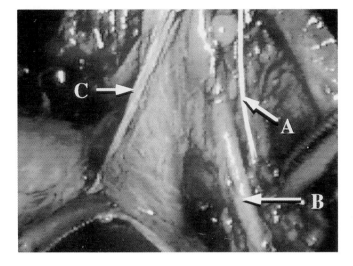 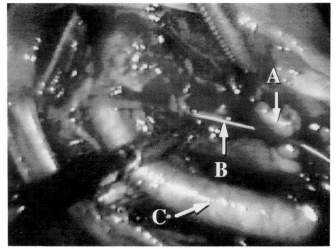

Figure 9-1 The right obturator nerve (A) can be exposed either by moving the external iliac artery (B) medially away from the psoas muscle or by dissecting posterior-laterally from the hypogastric artery (C).

Figure 9-2 Obturator lymph nodes (A) are elevated with care from the nerve (B) and removed using dissecting forceps while the external iliac artery (C) is retracted medially.

vein, and should be clipped and severed to prevent tearing. The dissection is complete when all nodes have been removed from the external iliac vessels, hypogastric artery, and obturator nerve and membrane. The region should be thoroughly irrigated and inspected for bleeding or for residual nodes. Because of magnification, the nodes and vessels can actually be seen better with the laparoscope than at open laparotomy, but the dissection is difficult and tedious (12).

The pelvic lymphadenectomy can also be done through a retroperitoneal approach (13). The retroperitoneal pelvic spaces are entered through a suprapubic incision. Blunt dissection lateral to the obliterated hypogastric artery opens the retroperitoneal region for dissection similar to that previously described. This approach has the advantage of avoiding the creation of intraperitoneal adhesions, but a disadvantage is the loss of intraperitoneal inspection unless it is done in conjunction with the node resection.

Para-aortic node biopsy

Para-aortic nodes are inspected by placing the patient in steep Trendelenburg position and gently brushing the bowel cephalad. The laparoscope is left in the umbilical position and the aorta and the proximal common iliac arteries are viewed directly posterior. Then, the vena cava and, laterally, the ureters should be located. With traction on the peritoneum over the aorta, the peritoneum is elevated and cut with just the tips of the scissors. It should be remembered that there is no depth perception and the most hazardous cut is in line and directly away from the scope. The surgeon uses the scissors in the right hand through the trocar just to the left of the scope and retracts with a grasping instrument through the left trocar; the assistant retracts with the right grasper as the para-aortic nodes are carefully removed. If bleeding occurs, small vessels are grasped and cauterized, or a vascular clip through a 10-mm trocar is used. Ties and suture are also available; if a large laceration should occur in a major vein, the positive intra-abdominal carbon dioxide pressure should be immediately reversed, and venous pressure increased with a fluid bolus and vasoconstriction while an incision is made to repair the laceration.

Laparoscopically assisted vaginal hysterectomy

In considering laparoscopically *assisted vaginal* hysterectomy (LAVH), we stress that this is an *assisted* vaginal hysterectomy. The purposes of the laparoscopic approach are to ensure removal of the ovaries and surgically stage the cancer (14,15). Cutting and suturing the inferior paracervical ligaments and uterine arteries have been performed safely for years through the vagina in performing vaginal hysterectomy, and to us, there appears to be no advantage in recommending a change that could put the ureters at possibly greater risk (16).

The LAVH is begun by inspecting the pelvis and identifying the ureters through the peritoneum. The peritoneum anterior (superior) to the ureter is cut just posterior to the ovary and infundibulopelvic ligament. A second incision is made immediately lateral and also parallel to the infundibulopelvic ligament. The latter incision is peforated by either starting with an incision through the round ligament using cautery set at 15–20 and extending the incision cephalad (usually without cautery for the peritoneum) or by starting cephalad over the psoas muscle and cutting toward the round ligament. The infundibulopelvic ligament is now isolated (Figure 9-3) and the ureter should be checked once more. The ligament is then cut 2–3 cm proximal to the ovary by using either an automatic stapling device, by securing it with individual ties, or with cautery (17). The ovaries may be left in place as well by securing and severing the ovarian ligament. Then, the ovaries should be secured to the peritoneum over the ileopsoas muscle by using a permanent suture. The ovaries can also be transposed, even as a part of staging laparoscopy without hysterectomy, if radiation therapy is anticipated (18); in

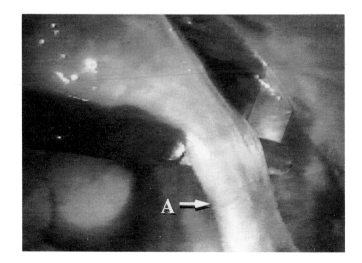

Figure 9-3 The right infundibulopelvic ligament is isolated and may be secured by one of several methods, including ligatures, cautery, or staples.

Figure 9-4 Peritoneum (A) of the
bladder (B) is incised over the cervix.

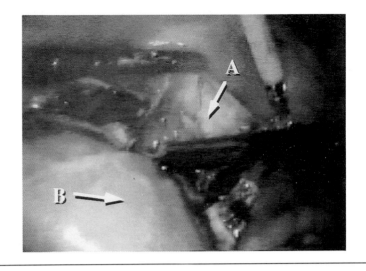

this case, the ovaries are marked with a radio-opaque clip. Ovaries are rarely involved with cervical cancer, particularly squamous cell carcinoma (19). The adnexa may be removed, of course, if a hysterectomy is not done by ligating the ovarian ligament after securing the infundibulopelvic.

The LAVH is continued by cutting the peritoneum of the bladder reflection over the cervix, thereby joining the incision of the round ligaments (Figure 9-4). The bladder is dissected down but only as far as is easily done, because this portion of the dissection will usually progress faster from below; the most important help is gained simply by cutting the peritoneum. Before turning to the vaginal portion of the hysterectomy, the peritoneum of the posterior cul-de-sac is cut to ensure that the rectum is free, and adhesions should also be cut.

Upon completion of the vaginal hysterectomy, the LAVH is concluded by returning to laparoscopic inspection for bleeding by carefully irrigating and looking at each point of surgery.

Radical hysterectomy via laparoscopy has also been described but is beyond the purpose of this review (20).

In summary, these laparoscopic procedures have demonstrated utility in the management of cervical carcinoma: intraperitoneal inspection, staging, peritoneal biopsy, pelvic and para-aortic node biopsy or lymphadenectomy, ovarian transposition, adnexectomy, and LAVH. We will now discuss a place for each of these in the care of cervical cancer.

Application of laparoscopy to specific situations

Preinvasive and microinvasive cancer

For preinvasive and microinvasive cervical cancer calling for hysterectomy, LAVH provides assistance in removing the ovaries. Laparoscopy can be particularly helpful if there is a synchronous pelvic mass that could be either a myoma or a primary ovarian tumor (21). For example, a woman with microinvasive cervical cancer and a large pelvic mass in which imaging could not distinguish a myoma from an ovarian neoplasm; laparoscopy readily determined it to be one large myoma and multiple smaller myomas. The infundibulopelvic ligaments were isolated and severed, and the steps previously described for LAVH and bilateral salpingo-oophorectomy (BSO) were followed. The uterus was then delivered from below with morcellation to complete the hysterectomy. Thus, the appropriate procedure was accomplished without an incision that would otherwise have been required.

Small IB and IIA cancers

For small cervical cancers exceeding microinvasion, an incision can also be avoided by laparoscopic pelvic lymphadenectomy and radical vaginal hysterectomy (22,23). The lymphadenectomy may be either transperitoneal or retroperitoneal. If the nodes are removed first and contain metastatic cancer, a decision to omit the hysterectomy and proceed with radiation therapy would be appropriate (10); in which case, avoiding an incision would be an advantage in minimizing the time before starting radiation therapy (24).

Inadvertant hysterectomy and invasive cancer, "cut-through"

If a hysterectomy has been done and a previously unrecognized invasive cancer discovered, i.e., so-called cut-through hysterectomy, the alternatives to treatment consist of either extended resection of the vaginal apex and lymphadenectomy (25), similar to radical hysterectomy, or radiation therapy. The latter avoids a second operation, but adhesions of bowel in the pelvis from the primary surgery can result in radiation bowel injury. Laparoscopy can be used to free the bowel and surgically stage the tumor; radiation can be started without delay immediately after laparoscopy.

Large central tumors, "barrel lesions"

Large stage IB and IIA cervical cancers over 4–5 cm in diameter, "barrel shaped" tumors, may be treated with abbreviated radiation and standard hysterectomy. Prior to initiating radiation, we have used laparoscopic staging particularly to exclude para-aortic (26) and occult peritoneal metastases. (If the para-aortic nodes are involved, extended field radiation can help as many as 28%.) Four to six weeks after radiation and brachytherapy, a hysterectomy by laparotomy or LAVH is done. Laparoscopic staging will not delay radiation treatment, which can be started on the first postoperative day, but radiation treatment and port size would be significantly altered if occult metastatic cancer is discovered.

Laparoscopy preceding radiation of large advanced stage cancer

Before starting radiation for advanced cancers, laparoscopy has had several uses: evaluation and removal of adnexal pathology, ovarian trans-

[117]

position, and surgical staging. Synchronous ovarian pathology, including endometriomas, inflammatory disease, and neoplasms (27,28,29,30), may be managed through laparoscopy. The adnexa are removed either through a trocar site that can be extended if necessary or through a colpotomy incision (31). Ovarian neoplasms, endometriosis, and chronically infected adnexa are, of course, better removed prior to starting radiation.

A third of large cervical cancers (clinical stages IIB, III, and IVA) have occult metastatic cancer outside the standard ports of radiation therapy; frequently, these are unrecognized by the best imaging methods. Laparoscopy may assist in staging, in freeing adhesions, and in transposing the ovaries, if desired.

We also do an incidental appendectomy through the laparoscope at the time of diagnostic and operative laparoscopy (32). If pain in the abdomen were to develop in the future, as it may with women having had complex treatment for cervical cancer, we would then not be concerned with the possibility of acute appendicitis.

When considering surgery, in every circumstance that radiation follows surgery in the sequence of treatment, we would anticipate that laparoscopy should enjoy a distinct advantage over laparotomy: there will likely be fewer adhesions in the proposed radiation field, and there should be a shorter delay required before starting radiation by avoiding an incision.

With difficult brachytherapy

Finally, we use laparoscopy to assist with difficult brachytherapy. Intraoperative pelvic ultrasound has been indispensable in the proper placement of the intrauterine tandem when obliteration of the cervical uterine canal by cancer or radiation fibrosis otherwise prevents safe placement of the tandem. On occasion, however, the ultrasound has been equivocal. In that event, direct laparoscopic inspection has been used to verify placement, but it has also shown the trocar to be in the peritoneal cavity more than once; the trocar was withdrawn and repositioned within the uterus while watching through the laparoscope.

In yet another type of brachytherapy using needles, laparoscopy has assisted with the iridium needles placement. For example, three women developing paravaginal recurrent cancer following radical hysterectomy received external radiation and brachytherapy using a Syed-Neblett template. Laparoscopic adhesiolysis freed bowel from fixation in the pelvis; the needles were then inserted with visual guidance to avoid bowel perforation by a needle or a needle being placed in the peritoneal cavity (Figure 9-5). On the other hand, adequate depth of needle placement was also assured.

Therefore, diagnostic and advanced operative laparoscopy has been helpful in the management of all stages and sizes of cervical cancer. The role of laparoscopy has been either through direct treatment or to assist with primary treatment, usually to refine radiation therapy. Ovarian

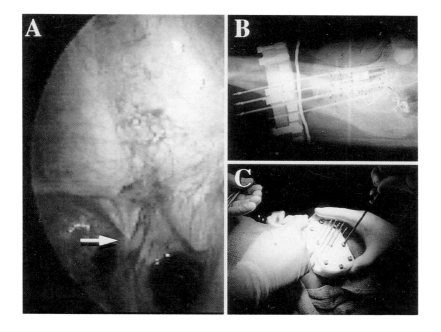

Figure 9-5 Laparoscopy guides the placement of a Syed needle application and also provides a means to free bowel that may have become fixed in the pelvis. (A) Needle elevates the peritoneum just to the right of the tip of the Foley catheter. (B) Lateral pelvic X-ray of the needles. (C) Needles are inserted through a template while the depth is checked through the laparoscope (A).

preservation or, when necessary, adnexectomy has been of additional benefit. Also, adhesiolysis may reduce the risk of radiation enteritis.

Complications

Complications of advanced laparoscopic procedures, extensive dissection and adhesiolysis, adnexectomy, lymphadenectomy, etc., include hemorrhage and injury to a viscus and ureter as well as infection, bowel obstruction, and hernia into a trocar site. Burn from electrocautery is a significant hazard. In addition, fatal CO_2 embolus through a laceration of a major vein is possible (33). Whether conversion to a laparotomy from laparoscopy should, of itself, be classified as a complication is questionable. If the preoperative surgical goals were safely and adequately attained in the majority of patients having laparoscopy, but laparotomy was required in the remainder to correct a problem or to achieve the surgical goal, the majority would still have been spared a laparotomy; the others would have had the laparotomy that would have been done regardless. Therefore, we do not consider conversion to laparotomy to be a complication, although it does need to be recorded; the reason to convert the procedure to a laparotomy should be noted and may itself be listed as a complication as would be any injury, whether or not it required a laparotomy for correction. Conversion certainly adds to the expense and operative time, although experience should reduce the conversion rate through enhanced laparoscopy skills and improved case selection.

Incidence and prevention of complications

The actual rate of complications reported by seven French referral centers was favorable (34). One death in 17,521 procedures was reported.

[119]

The rates of nonlethal complications were 1.1/1000 diagnostic and minor procedures and 5.2/1000 major and advanced procedures. Also, the laparotomy rate was 0.5–1.17/1000 diagnostic and minor procedures as compared to 8.4–8.9/1000 major and advanced procedures. Visceral complications in 40 and hemorrhage in 17 were the most frequently reported.

Experience and strict observance of proper technique will minimize problems (35). Yet, a lack of depth perception, of tactile sensation, and of a wide field of view are limitations currently inherent to operative laparoscopy. To a much greater degree than with laparotomy, the operator is dependent on a number of sophisticated instruments and upon a skilled support staff. Therefore, a number of malfunctions that could cause a complication exist and may occur even without the operator's knowledge. In addition, the potential for fatal CO_2 embolus associated with dissection around large veins is particularly worrisome. Electrical injuries also continue to be a hazard (36).

Because many oncology patients will have had radiation or prior surgery and because bowel and vascular injuries are encountered with sharp entry of the primary trocar or needle, we prefer to use an open method with the blunt port (37,38).

Cautery burns are minimized by taking several precautions: (1) disconnecting the cautery from the instrument except when in use, (2) removing instruments of any type when they are not being used, (3) seeing completely around and beyond any tissue being cauterized, (4) keeping the warning sound of the cautery unit on high volume to avoid inadvertent cautery (a problem also unlikely if the cautery is disconnected except when in immediate use), and (5) using the lowest effective setting. We also prefer to use clips rather than cautery when working near bowel.

Summary

The preceding survey describes applications of laparoscopy in the management of cervical cancer broadly defined for (1) surgical staging and planning of subsequent treatment, (2) recognition and management of synchronous pathology, (3) adhesiolysis to free bowel, (4) preservation of ovarian function, (5) assisting difficult brachytherapy, (6) lymphadenectomy, and (7) LAVH. We have experience with all and have had enthusiasm for para-aortic and pelvic lymphadenectomy; however, the concern for gaseous embolism as well as the skill required for these two procedures demand caution. In our opinion, applications 1, 2, 3, 4, and 5 will likely prove to be the most lasting, while para-aortic and pelvic lymphadenectomy will likely remain, at least for a while, in the hands of those with special interest in this area.

References

1 American Cancer Society. 1991 facts & figures. Atlanta, American Cancer Society, 1991.

[120]

2 Beahrs OH, Henson DE, Hutter RVP, Myers MH, eds. Manual for staging of cancer, 3rd ed. Philadelphia: JB Lippincott, 1988:151–153.

3 Photopulos GJ, Vander Zwagg R. Class II radical hysterectomy shows less morbidity and good treatment efficacy compared to class III. Gynecol Oncol 1991;40:21–24.

4 Photopulos GJ. Surgery or radiation for early cervical cancer. Clin Obstet Gynecol 1990;33:872–882.

5 Maruyama Y, van Nagell JR, Yoneda J, et al. Dose-response failure pattern for bulky or barrel-shaped stage IB cervical cancer treated by combined photon irradiation and extrafascial hysterectomy. Cancer 1989;63:70–76.

6 O'Quinn AG, Fletcher GH, Wharton JT. Guidelines for conservative hysterectomy after irradiation. Gynecol Oncol 1980;9:68–79.

7 Touboul E, Lefranc JP, Blondon J, et al. Preoperative radiation therapy and surgery in the treatment of "bulky" squamous cell carcinoma of the uterine cervix (stage Ib, IIa, and IIb operable tumors). Radiother Oncol 1992;24:32–40.

8 Weiser EB, Bundy BN, Hoskins WJ, et al. Extraperitoneal versus transperitoneal selective para-aortic lymphadenectomy in the pretreatment surgical staging of advanced cervical carcinoma (Gynecologic Oncology Group study). Gynecol Oncol 1989;33:283–289.

9 Welander CE, Pierce VK, Nordi D, et al. Pretreatment laparotomy in carcinoma of the cervix. Gynecol Oncol 1981;12:336–347.

10 Childers JM, Hatch K, Surwit EA. The role of laparoscopic lymphadenectomy in the management of cervical carcinoma. Gynecol Oncol 1992;47:38–43.

11 Taillandier J, Boiteux JP, Giraud B. Pelvic lymphadenoscopy. A simple reliable method for the staging of pelvic cancers. Int Surg 1992;77:208–210.

12 Querleu D, Leblanc E, Castelain B. Laparoscopic pelvic lymphadenectomy in the staging of early carcinoma of the cervix. Am J Obstet Gynecol 1991;164:579–581.

13 Dargent D, Arnould P. Percutaneous pelvic lymphadenectomy under laparoscopic guidance. In: Nichols D, ed. Gynecologic and obstetric surgery. St. Louis: Mosby Year Book, Inc. 1993:583–605.

14 Mage G, Wattiez A, Chapron C, Canis M, Pouly JL, Pingeon JM, Bruhat MA. Laparoscopic hysterectomy. Results in 44 cases. J Gynecol Obstet Biol Reprod 1992;21:436–444.

15 Nezhat F, Nezhat C, Gordon S, Wilkins E. Laparoscopic versus abdominal hysterectomy. J Reprod Med 1992;37:247–250.

16 Woodland MB. Ureter injury during laparoscopy-assisted vaginal hysterectomy with the endoscopic linear stapler. Am J Obstet Gynecol 1992;756–757.

17 Daniel JF, Kurtz BR, Lee JY. Laparoscopic oophorectomy: comparative study of ligatures, bipolar coagulation, and automatic stapling devices. Obstet Gynecol 1992;80:325–328.

18 Prouvost MA, Canis M, Le Bouedec G, et al. Ovarian transposition with percelioscopy before curietherapy in stage IA and IB cancer of the uterine cervix. J Gynecol Obstet Biol Reprod 1991;20:361–365.

19 Toki N, Tsukamoto N, Kaku T, et al. Microscopic ovarian metastasis of the uterine cervical cancer. Gynecol Oncol 1991;41:46–51.

20 Nezhat CR, Burrell MO, Nezhat FR, Benigo BB, Welander CE. Laparoscopic radical hysterectomy with paraaortic and pelvic node dissection. Am J Obstet Gynecol 1992;66:864–865.

21 Maher PJ, Wood EC, Hill DJ, et al. Laparoscopically assisted hysterectomy. Med J Aust 1992;156:316–318.

22 Zhang QB. Vaginal radical hysterectomy for uterine cervical cancer. Chin Med J 1990;103:743–747.

23 Dargent D, Mathevet P. Radical laparoscopic vaginal hysterectomy. J Gynecol Obstet Biol Reprod 1992;21:709–710.

24 Vigliotti AP, Wen BC, Hussey DH, Doornbos JF, Staples JJ, et al. Extended field irradiation for carcinoma of the uterine cervix with positive periaortic nodes. Int J Radiat Oncol Biol Phys 1992;23:501–509.

25 Herd J, Fowler JM, Shenson D, et al. Laparoscopic para-aortic lymph node sampling: development of a technique. Gynecol Oncol 1992;44:271–276.

26 Ayhan A, Kucukozkan T, Tuncer ZS. Management of invasive cervical cancer in patients initially treated by simple hysterectomy. Eur J Surg Oncol 1992;18:177–179.

27 Nezhat C, Nezhat F, Burrell M. Laparoscopically-assisted hysterectomy for the man-

agement of a borderline ovarian tumor: a case report. J Laparoendosc Surg 1992;2:167–169.

28 Reich H, McGlynn F, Wilkie W. Laparoscopic management of stage I ovarian cancer. A case report. J Reprod Med 1990;35:601–604.

29 Hulka JF, Parker WH, Surrey MW, Phillips JM. Management of ovarian masses. AAGL 1990 Survey. 1992;37:599–602.

30 Cristalli B, Cayol A, Izard V, et al. Benefit of operative laparoscopy for ovarian tumors suspected of benignity. J Laparoendosc Surg 1992;2:69–73.

31 Wood C, Hill D, Maher P, et al. Laparoscopic adnexectomy—indicators, technique and results. Aust N Z J Obstet Gynaecol 1992;32:362–366.

32 Wolenski M, Markus E, Pelosi MA. Laparoscopic appendectomy incidental to gynecologic procedures. Today's OR Nurse 1991;13:12–18.

33 Duncan C. Carbon dioxide embolism during laparoscopy: a case report. AANA J 1992;60:139–144.

34 Querleu D, Chapron C, Chevallier L, et al. Complications of gynecologic laparoscopic surgery–a French multicenter collaborative study. New Engl J Med Surg 1993; 328:1355.

35 Aubriot FX. Techniques: advantages, complications, contraindications. Rev Prat 1991;41:2541–2545.

36 Lehmann-Willenbrock E, Riedel HH, Mecke H, et al. Pelviscopy/laparoscopy and its complications in Germany, 1949–1988. J Reprod Med 1992;37:671–677.

37 Oshinsky GS, Smith AD. Laparoscopic needles and trocars: an overview of designs and complications. J Laparoendosc Surg 1992;2:117–125.

38 Tews G, Bohaumilitzky T, Arzt W, et al. Decreasing the surgical risk of laparoscopy by using a newly developed, blunt trocar. Geburtshilfe Frauennheilkd 1991;51:304–306.

10   Laparoscopic Approaches to Uterine Malignancy for Endometrial Cancer

JOEL M. CHILDERS

Since the turn of the century, physicians have known that most women with early endometrial carcinoma can be cured by hysterectomy and removal of the adnexa. Abdominal hysterectomy has been the technique most frequently employed. In fact, in 1900, Thomas Cullen recommended this as the treatment of choice for patients with endometrial carcinoma (1). A brief historical overview is important in understanding why laparoscopy may play a significant role in the management of endometrial cancer patients in the future.

From clinical to surgical-pathological staging

It has been recognized for a number of years that patients with early disease and/or well-differentiated lesions have done better than patients with more advanced disease and/or less differentiated lesions. Unfortunately, early literature on survival rates did not differentiate for such factors as grade of the tumor or depth of myometrial invasion. As survival data became available, investigators noted a clear relationship between survival and differentiation of tumor (2).

Individual investigators and literature reviews have also indicated that the survival of patients with endometrial carcinoma decreased as myometrial invasion increased (2). Cheon reported an increased percentage of deep myometrial invasion with decreased differentiation of tumor (3). Creasman et al. demonstrated, by surgical staging, a higher percentage of lymph node involvement, both pelvic and para-aortic, with increasing grade and depth of myometrial invasion (4). Following this, the Gynecologic Oncology Group (GOG) initiated prospective surgical-pathological studies in clinical stage I subjects. This group's original limited institutional study, as well as the group-wide study involving 621 patients with clinical stage I carcinoma of the endometrium, substantiated the previously reported relationships between grade of tumor and depth of myometrial invasion (5,6). In addition, the correlation between pelvic and para-aortic lymph node metastases and tumor grade and depth of invasion were verified. It was also noted that as the depth of invasion increased within each grade category, so did the chances of lymph node metastases.

Surgical-pathological staging studies have clearly demonstrated the inaccuracies of clinical staging (4–11). Because clinical evaluation is

[123]

unable to identify most adnexal metastases, intraperitoneal implants, and nodal metastases, 15% to 28% of patients with clinical stage I endometrial carcinoma are understaged. Since, grade for grade, survival rates did not seem to be affected by whether the patient had received preoperative radium and surgery or surgery alone (12–14), and since potential important prognostic factors, such as depth of invasion, vascular space invasion, true tumor grade, peritoneal cytology, estrogen-progesterone receptor status, and DNA ploidy are potentially unevaluable in patients who have received preoperative radiotherapy, surgical-pathological staging made sound scientific sense. Realizing clinical staging was potentially quite inaccurate when treatment results were analyzed, the cancer committee of the International Federation of Gynecology and Obstetrics (FIGO) changed their classification for endometrial carcinoma from a clinical to a surgical-pathological staged disease (15). For all of these reasons, the once common practice of administering preoperative radiation therapy to patients with endometrial carcinoma has now largely been abandoned for primary surgical-pathological staging.

Vaginal hysterectomy in endometrial cancer

Believing survival could be compromised, the use of vaginal hysterectomy by physicians treating patients with adenocarcinoma of the endometrium has been limited. This approach to patients with endometrial cancer has been documented for several decades by the Europeans. Bastiaanse, in a retrospective study of 217 patients, reported on the use of total vaginal hysterectomy to treat patients with all stages and grades of endometrial carcinoma (16). This study, which was published in 1952, reported a survival rate of 72%. This uncorrected survival rate is similar to the 73% survival rate reported by Ingiulla and Cosmi in their retrospective study of 112 patients treated with total vaginal hysterectomy and bilateral salpingo-oophorectomy (BSO) (17). They too treated patients of all stages and grades.

The largest American experience using vaginal hysterectomy to treat patients with endometrial cancer has been at the Mayo Clinic (18–21). In four separate reports that cover the years from 1930 to 1972, with very little overlap, they mention the use of total vaginal hysterectomy in 263 patients. The first of these publications (18) reports a five-year survival of 82.7% (67/81). The second report, and the only publication from this institution devoted solely to the use of vaginal hysterectomy, is also the largest American series on this approach to endometrial cancer (19). This retrospective study of 100 patients comprised 15% (100/659) of the patients with endometrial cancer treated at the Mayo Clinic during the decade 1945–1954. The vaginal approach was used in only 44 patients for medical reasons. Forty-three of these patients had ovaries that, for technical reasons, were not removed. In this publication, Pratt et al. reported an 89% corrected five-year survival (95% for grade 1 tumors and 72.7% for grade 3 tumors). Three patients required morcellation of the uterus; none of these three died of disease. In four of the ten patients who died of disease within five years, ovaries had been left behind.

The most recent report from the Mayo Clinic confirms this five-year survival rate (21). In the report by Malkasian et al. on the management of patients with endometrial cancer between 1962 and 1972, 67 patients were treated by total vaginal hysterectomy. The five-year survival for these patients with grade 2 and 3 tumors did not differ from that of patients treated with abdominal hysterectomy, and the outcome for patients with well-differentiated tumors was higher than predicted by the actuarial tables.

This similarity in five-year survival rate between patients with stage I endometrial carcinoma treated with total vaginal hysterectomy and those treated with total abdominal hysterectomy (TAH) is confirmed in a report by Candiani et al. (22) They reported on 425 patients treated in the decade between 1970 and 1980 using three different surgical approaches: TAH with BSO and selective pelvic lymphadenectomy (245 patients), TAH and BSO (100 patients), and total vaginal hysterectomy with BSO (80 patients). A similar corrected five-year survival rate was observed in each of these three groups (81%, 90%, and 88%, respectively). Unfortunately, the number of grade 2 and 3 lesions was not evenly distributed (69%, 35%, and 43%, respectively), and, therefore, sound conclusions concerning survival and surgical approach cannot be reached.

The current literature reflects the limited use of vaginal hysterectomy for the treatment of patients with endometrial carcinoma. There are only three reports in the American literature on this topic in the last ten years. The report by Candiani et al. is the only one of these publications that did not limit this surgical approach to medically compromised patients (22). It is also the only European report. The remaining two publications are both retrospective American studies addressing the use of vaginal hysterectomy for the management of medically compromised patients with stage I endometrial cancer.

Peters et al. combined experiences from the University of Virginia and the University of Michigan over the 27 years from 1955 through 1981 (23). Vaginal hysterectomy was performed in 56 patients because of obesity or major medical problems. The five-year survival for all patients was 94%. The five-year survival was 98% with grade 1 tumors, 78% with grade 2 tumors, and 84% with grade 3 tumors. In only 10 of the patients (18%) in this group were the adnexa removed. Thirty-two patients received adjuvant radiotherapy.

Several of the surgical techniques discussed in this report deserve mention. These authors are the first to describe procurement of pelvic washings upon entering the cul-de-sac. While the clinical significance of malignant peritoneal cytology in patients with early endometrial carcinoma has not been completely defined and is certainly beyond the scope of this chapter, most investigators believe that this information is worth retrieving (24). To assist in removal of the uterus, they used Schuchardt's incisions in five patients and uterine morcellation in seven. Six patients in this latter group had grade 1 tumors while one had a grade 3 tumor.

Bloss et al. reported the only other recently published American experience (25). They combined the experience of three institutions over the 20 years from 1970 to 1990. All 31 of their patients had clinical stage I endometrial carcinoma and were treated with total vaginal hysterectomy because they were considered to be at high risk for morbidity and mortality from an abdominal approach. Risk factors included morbid obesity, hypertension, diabetes mellitus, and cardiovascular disease. Thirty-five percent of their patients received adjuvant radiotherapy because of deep myometrial invasion or unfavorable histology. There was only one cancer-related death, which occured 4½ years following surgery in a patient with a poorly differentiated lesion, resulting in a 93% five-year survival rate. Three patients experienced serious postoperative complications that extended their hospitalizations (hemorrhage requiring abdominal exploration, pulmonary embolism, and myocardial infarction). There were no postoperative deaths.

Those authors have several recommendations for safely accomplishing vaginal hysterectomies in these patients. Episiotomy (either unilateral or bilateral) and suturing the labia to the inner thighs is recommended to improve exposure. The authors recommend preoperative ultrasound assessment to identify large uteri, which may help avoid morcellation of the uterus, a technique which they do not recommend and was not used in any of the patients in their series. While removal of the adnexa was recommended and was performed in 11 (35%) of their patients, they did not believe that failure to do so warranted abdominal exploration.

While these authors did not comment on the ability to procure pelvic washings in this retrospective study, they did point out that a major objection to vaginal surgery in the treatment of endometrial carcinoma is the inability to assess pelvic lymph nodes and extrauterine disease as well as to guarantee removal of the adnexa. Pratt et al. pointed out that adnexal disease, either neoplastic or inflammatory, or a uterus that is fixed high in the pelvis by inflammation or endometriosis, are further drawbacks to the vaginal approach (19).

Rationale for laparoscopy in endometrial cancer

Laparoscopically assisted hysterectomy and laparoscopic lymphadenectomy are both recently reported techniques. Since the report of Reich et al. on laparoscopic hysterectomy, several reports of series of patients have followed (26–31). While these studies are all limited to benign disease, they report on the use of the laparoscope to convert an abdominal procedure to a vaginal procedure. Initial reports on laparoscopic lymphadenectomy were limited to pelvic lymph nodes (32–34). However, laparoscopic removal of para-aortic lymph nodes soon became feasible (35), and shortly thereafter, these three techniques (hysterectomy and pelvic and para-aortic lymphadenectomy) were combined for the management of patients with stage I endometrial carcinoma (36). Laparoscopy was used to (a) assess the intraperitoneal cavity, (b) obtain washings, (c) guarantee removal of the adnexa, (d) perform pelvic and para-aortic lymph node sampling, and (e) guarantee vaginal removal of the uterus.

[126]

Believing operative laparoscopy could overcome the surgical limitations of the pure vaginal approach in patients with clinical stage I endometrial carcinoma, we prospectively studied the role of laparoscopically assisted surgical staging (LASS) in these patients to determine the feasibility, safety, limiting factors, and advantages of this approach in patients with clinical stage I disease.

Patients and preoperative considerations

Our first 61 patients who were considered candidates for LASS to manage their clinical stage I endometrial carcinoma were chosen over a two-year period between May 1991 and May 1993. Their ages ranged from 40 to 85 years, with a mean of 69; 41% (24/59) were > 71 years of age. Their weights ranged from 102 to 298 pounds, with a mean of 153; 21% (12/59) were > 179 pounds.

Preoperatively, all patients underwent complete history and physical examinations and routine laboratory investigation, including chest x-ray, electrocardiogram, and complete blood count. All patients were counseled regarding the investigational nature of this surgical staging procedure. Each patient received a mechanical bowel preparation consisting of two days of clear liquids and 240 cc of magnesium citrate/day for two days prior to surgery.

All procedures were performed at one of three local hospitals, and in all cases, laparoscopic videocameras were used; however, at each institution different telescopes, cameras, light sources, insufflators, and instruments were utilized. All patients were admitted the morning of surgery, and the procedures were performed using general anesthesia. Each patient was placed in the dorsal lithotomy position, extending the upper legs as much as possible in order to keep the knees away from the abdomen. Prophylactic antibiotics were administered preoperatively. The patients' arms were tucked by their sides with padding used over the ulnar nerve. A uterine manipulator was inserted after the patient was prepared and draped in the standard sterile fashion.

The LASS schema

Our current algorithm for the management of patients with clinical stage I adenocarcinoma of the endometrium includes selective laparoscopic lymph node sampling based upon grade of tumor, depth of invasion, and the presence of extrauterine disease (Figure 10-1). Patients with well-differentiated lesions have LAVH first, while patients with grade 2 or 3

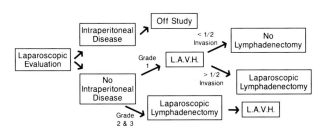

Figure 10-1 Schema for laparoscopic assisted surgical staging (LASS) of patients with clinical stage I endometrial carcinoma.

[127]

lesions undergo lymphadenectomy prior to the hysterectomy. Patients with well-differentiated lesions invading greater than one half of the myometrium, as determined by frozen section, undergo laparoscopic lymphadenectomy. All lymphadenectomies are bilateral, including the para-aortic lymph node sampling, thus adhering to the current GOG surgical procedure manual (37). Before we had developed the technique of left-sided para-aortic lymphadenectomy, a right-sided-only sampling was performed (38).

The operative technique

Instrument insertion

We insert the 10-mm disposable primary trocar directly into the intraperitoneal cavity without creating a pneumoperitoneum. This is accomplished after making an incision in the umbilicus and applying upward traction on the anterior abdominal wall with the aid of towel clips placed on either side of the umbilicus. The telescope verifies intraperitoneal placement prior to beginning insufflation. We believe this technique is safe and faster than insufflating with the Veress needle. It also avoids the annoying preperitoneal insufflation that can occur.

In patients with umbilical hernias or previous abdominal incisions extending to or through the umbilicus, we use the left upper quadrant (39). First, a Veress needle is placed in the ninth intercostal space between the midclavicular line and the midaxillary line. A 5-mm disposable trocar is then inserted, after insufflation, approximately 1 cm below the costal margin lateral to the superior epigastric vessels. This port is then used to assess the intraperitoneal cavity for adhesions and for safe sites for placement of additional trocars.

Four laparoscopic ports are used to perform the LASS procedure. The primary (camera) port is in the umbilicus and is 10 mm. Two 5-mm ports are placed lateral to the epigastric vessels approximately midway between the umbilicus and the anterior superior iliac spine bilaterally (Figure 10-2). The fourth port is placed in the midline above the pubic symphysis and is 10 or 11 mm. Additional port sites for para-aortic lymphadenectomy have been suggested but have been infrequently used in our procedures (40,41). Screw-in fascial anchors are not used, but each sleeve is anchored to the skin with a silk suture. This does not enlarge the fascial defect and allows the sleeve to be inserted farther into the abdominal cavity, but prevents it from being pulled out of the abdominal cavity.

Inspection of the intraperitoneal cavity

After the laparoscopic ports are placed, the intraperitoneal cavity is inspected systematically in a clockwise fashion. The pelvis is evaluated only after the establishment of Trendelenburg position. Cul-de-sac fluid and/or pelvic washings are then taken and the area from the duodenum to the lower pelvis is inspected for obvious adenopathy.

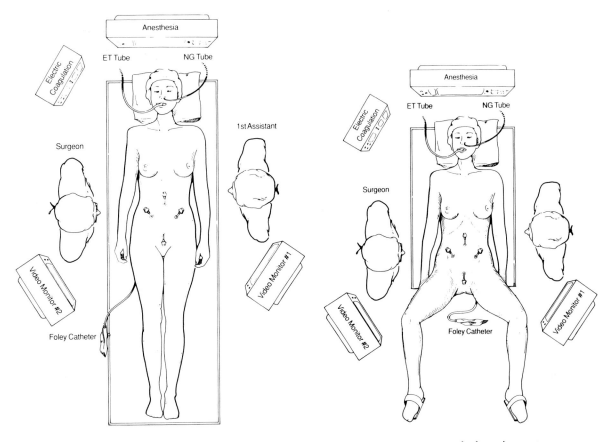

Figure 10-2 The operating room setup is illustrated in this figure. Four trocars are used; the primary trocar (camera port) is in the umbilicus and the three ancillary trocars are in the lower abdomen. Two 5-mm ports are placed lateral to the inferior epigastric vessels and a 10-mm or larger port is placed in the midline suprapubically. Note that two monitors are being used, which is necessary for the para-aortic lymph node sampling. The dorsal lithotomy position is used but not illustrated here.

Pelvic lymphadenectomy

To perform a laparoscopic pelvic or para-aortic lymphadenectomy, the surgeon stands on the side opposite the nodes to be dissected. The assistant controls the telescope in the umbilical port and a grasper placed through the ipsilateral lateral port. The surgeon uses a grasper through the lower midline port and scissors with monopolar cautery capability through the contralateral lateral port.

The retroperitoneal space is entered by transecting the round ligament using monopolar electrocautery (Plate 12). The broad ligament is opened and the obliterated umbilical artery is identified near the bladder and retracted medially (Plate 13). This potential space between the obliterated umbilical artery and the external iliac vein is easily opened and allows prompt identification of the obturator nerve. The nodal and fatty tissue along the anterior aspect of this nerve is dissected by blunt and sharp dissection.

Next, the nodal and fatty tissue along the medial aspect of the external iliac vein is dissected off this vein by blunt and sharp dissection (Plate 14). Care is taken to avoid inadvertent damage to aberrant or accessory veins in this area.

[129]

The nodal bundle is then transected at the pelvic wall using monopolar electricity. The only remaining attachment of the obturator nodal package is at the bifurcation of the hypogastric and external iliac arteries. Transection in this area is accomplished carefully by blunt dissection and judicious use of monopolar electricity. The nodal bundle is removed through the lower 10-mm suprapubic port. We do not concern ourselves at this time with meticulous removal of the nodes at the bifurcation of the common iliac artery. We have found it easier to accomplish this after the external and low common iliac nodes have been removed.

External iliac lymph node sampling is accomplished by first identifying the genitofemoral nerve on the psoas muscle (Plate 15). The nodal and fatty tissue medial to this nerve are removed by sharply dissecting in the adventitial plane of the external iliac artery. This dissection extends from the circumflex iliac artery to the distal common iliac artery. To avoid damaging the ureter and ovarian vessels when working over the common iliac artery, it is necessary for the assistant to retract these vessels in a cephalad direction. After this is accomplished, any remaining nodal tissue is dissected at the bifurcation of the common iliac artery (Plates 16, 17, 18). The proximal common iliac nodal tissue is removed during the para-aortic node sampling.

Laparoscopic para-aortic lymphadenectomy

Proper placement of the small bowel into the upper abdomen is paramount for exposure to the para-aortic area. The mesentery of the small bowel should be splayed out across the abdomen with the bowel in the upper abdomen. Trendelenburg position, a good bowel preparation, and, occasionally, lateral tilt of the operating table all assist in proper placement of the bowel in the upper abdomen. Depending on its location, the transverse duodenum may be visualized as it crosses the vena cava and aorta. The aorta, right common iliac artery, and the right ureter as it crosses the right iliac vessels should be located prior to beginning the para-aortic dissection. The camera is rotated 90° so that the aorta and vena cava are horizontal on the color monitor and the primary surgeon is oriented.

Using scissors, an incision is made in the peritoneum over the aorta and extended down the right common iliac toward the ureter and up the aorta to the mesentery of the small bowel or the transverse duodenum. The peritoneum is lifted with graspers and blunt dissection is performed laterally toward the psoas muscle. The right ureter is identified, dissected under, and lifted off the underlying psoas muscle bluntly. Blunt dissection is continued until the right psoas muscle and its tendon are visually identified.

The assistant places his grasper (in the right lateral port) beneath the ureter and retracts the ureter anteriorly and laterally out of the operative field. This retraction keeps the ureter out of the operative field and also creates a small "tent" that helps prevent small bowel from falling into the operative field.

The surgeon then dissects sharply in the adventitial plane of the aorta and right common iliac artery. Small vessels, both vascular and lymphatic, are coagulated with the tip of the scissors. Only after the aortic adventitia is cleaned off does lateral dissection begin. This un-roofing of the vena cava is carefully extended in a cephalad and caudad direction, avoiding inadvertent laceration of perforating vessels. Small perforating vessels are easily coagulated with the scissors. Large perfo-rating vessels may need to be clipped. We have used Endo-Clips (U.S. Surgical Corp., Norwalk, CT) placed through the 10-mm port in the lower midline. Generally, clips are not required because the majority of perforating vessels can be controlled with monopolar electrocautery.

One end of the nodal bundle is then transected. Whether one tran-sects the distal end near the right common iliac artery first or the cephalad end near the transverse duodenum is a matter of choice. This is accomplished by using monopolar coagulation. Once both ends of the nodal bundle are transected, the nodal package is extracted through the lower midline port. The operative field is irrigated and evaluated for hemostasis.

Left-sided para-aortic lymphadenectomy

The camera is rotated so that the aorta and the vena cava are horizontal on the color monitor and oriented for the surgeon on the right side of the patient. This will be 180° different in orientation from the right-sided sampling.

The dissection continues in adventitial planes previously created. This endopelvic fascia is dissected from the lower aorta and upper left common iliac artery. The cephalad extent of the dissection is limited by the inferior mesenteric artery.

After the adventitia over these vessels is dissected free, lateral dissec-tion toward the left psoas muscle is performed bluntly. The surgeon dissects beneath the left ureter and the mesentery of the rectosigmoid laterally until the psoas muscle and its tendon are identified. The assistant places his instrument into the dissected space beneath the mesentery of the rectosigmoid and the left ureter. This retraction is necessary for ade-quate exposure and protection of the ureter.

The nodal bundle is grasped and lifted anteriorly so the surgeon can dissect between this lymphatic chain and the aorta. Transection of the bundle is accomplished by monopolar electrocautery at the distal end first. The nodal chain lateral to the left common iliac artery up to the inferior mesenteric artery can be removed in toto. The proximal end near the inferior mesenteric artery is transected last. The specimen is removed through the lower midline 10-mm port, and the operative field is irrigated and inspected for hemostasis. No peritoneal closures are performed and no retroperitoneal drains are placed.

Laparoscopically assisted vaginal hysterectomy

The laparoscopically assisted vaginal hysterectomy is performed either before or after the laparoscopic lymphadenectomy, depending upon

[131]

grade of tumor and depth of myometrial invasion. If the lymphadenectomy has not been performed, the round ligaments are grasped and traction is applied with two grasping instruments. The tip of the scissors transect the round ligament, using monopolar coagulation (Plate 12). The round ligament is transected near the pelvic sidewall and the broad ligament is opened by applying medial traction to the transected round ligament. The ureter and ovarian vessels are identified on the medial leaf of the broad ligament, and a window is created between these two structures by sharp dissection with the scissors (Plate 19). The window is enlarged by sharp or blunt dissection, and a 2-0 or 0 silk suture is passed through the ipsilateral lateral port through the window, around the ovarian vessels, and back out through the port. This vascular pedicle is then ligated extracorporeally, using a Clarke knot pusher (Plate 20). A prefabricated chromic slipknot is placed through the ipsilateral lateral port and a grasper is placed through the slipknot prior to grasping the infundibulopelvic ligament distal to the silk ligature (Plate 21). The ovarian vessels are cut with scissors between the grasper and a silk suture. The slipknot is slipped around the grasper and over the infundibulopelvic ligament to backtie the pedicle. Another prefabricated slipknot is placed through the ipsilateral port, and the proximal end of the infundibulopelvic ligament is ligated, leaving the live end doubly ligated. The uterine manipulator shifts the corpus to one side to allow dissection of the broad ligament and skeletonization of the uterine arteries on the opposite side. The bladder flap is created by sharp dissection with the scissors.

The uterine vessels are transected only if it is felt they could not be easily clamped and suture-ligated from below. If laparoscopic ligation of the uterine arteries needs to be performed, it is done either with the Kleppinger bipolar forceps or by using the same suturing technique described on the infundibulopelvic ligament. In the latter instance, a prefabricated slipknot is placed into the abdomen through the suprapubic port; a grasper placed through the ipsilateral lateral port is placed through this slipknot, and the uterine artery and vein are grasped in a similar fashion as would be performed using a Heaney clamp during an abdominal procedure (Plate 22). The vessels are transected by sharp dissection and the loop is passed over the vessels and behind the grasper (Plate 23).

If the surgeon desires, a posterior colpotomy can be easily performed by using the disposable trocar (used umbilically) without its sleeve (42). The trocar is placed into the vagina and the colpotomy site selected by hugging the cervix and staying in the midline between the uterosacral ligaments. Under direct laparoscopic visualization, the protective sleeve is permitted to retract, allowing the trocar to enter the cul-de-sac (Plate 24). The trocar is removed and ring forceps are placed through the colpotomy incision and the incision extended bluntly by opening the ring forceps. This requires only a few moments and allows for easy placement of a weighted speculum into the cul-de-sac. The remainder of the procedure is performed vaginally. Thus far, we have not transected the cardinal or uterosacral ligaments laparoscopically.

We close the vaginal cuff with figure-eight sutures in a horizontal fashion and do not close the peritoneum. After completion of the hysterectomy, the abdomen is reinsufflated and the operative field inspected for hemostasis. No retroperitoneal drains are placed.

Results

Laparoscopic evaluation was performed on all 61 patients; six were discovered to have intraperitoneal disease. Of the remaining 55, we performed laparoscopic lymphadenectomy on 30 patients. Of the 25 patients who did not have lymph nodes sampled, all were at "low risk" for nodal involvement (stage IA grade 1 and stage IB grade 1) except for three patients. One of these three would consent only to hysterectomy and BSO, refusing lymphadenectomy, and postoperatively, she refused radiotherapy for her stage IC grade 1 lesion. We were unable to perform laparoscopic common iliac and para-aortic lymphadenectomies in the other two patients because of obesity. One patient with stage IC grade 1 carcinoma weighed 180 lbs., while the other patient, with a stage IB grade 2 lesion, weighed 250 lbs.

Of the 30 patients undergoing laparoscopic lymphadenectomy, one patient had right-sided para-aortic nodes positive for metastatic disease, and negative left-sided para-aortic nodes. Her lesion was poorly differentiated and deeply invasive.

Eight patients had grade 3 lesions and all were invasive. Of these, four had metastasized: one to the para-aortic nodes, one to the pelvic peritoneum and ovary, one to the abdominal peritoneum and omentum, and one to the right hemidiaphragm. The remaining four patients had stage I disease after LASS and laparoscopic lymphadenectomy. Fourteen patients had grade 2 lesions; ten were invasive, and three had metastasized, all to the pelvic peritoneum. None of the well-differentiated lesions had metastasized.

A total of eight patients had extrauterine disease: six intraperitoneal and two retroperitoneal. The disease was limited to the pelvis in four of the six patients with intraperitoneal disease, while two patients had upper abdominal disease. All metastatic lesions were less than 1 cm in size except for a solitary 2-cm right hemidiaphragm lesion. None of the metastases were predicted by preoperative evaluation.

Excluding the patients with extrauterine disease, one patient had positive washings. This patient had a stage Ia grade 1 lesion and was diagnosed preoperatively by hysteroscopy before referral to our practice. Since we believed this could be "contamination" secondary to hysteroscopy, we elected to perform diagnostic laparoscopy and washings 12 weeks posthysterectomy. Pelvic washings retrieved at the time of that procedure revealed no malignant cells.

All patients underwent LAVH except for two. The first had a laparoscopic bilateral pelvic and para-aortic lymphadenectomy and the ovarian vessels were transected. A small Pfannenstiel's incision was then made and abdominal hysterectomy was performed. She was nulliparous and had an 8-cm intramural fibroid. Abdominal wall retractors were not used and the bowel was not packed. She was discharged on postoperative day 2. The second patient is discussed under "Complications."

An additional patient had a pedunculated uterine leiomyoma of significant size, 6 cm in diameter. It was easily transected laparoscopically, using suture and electrocautery, prior to hysterectomy. Removal was accomplished vaginally after the uterus and adnexa were removed.

Complications

Three patients had significant complications. In one 65-year-old patient weighing 162 lbs., the left ureter was transected during ligation of the uterine artery using the Endo-GIA (United States Surgical Corp.). She was the ninth patient in our series and had had five previous laparotomies, including a diverting colostomy for ruptured diverticulitis and subsequent colostomy takedown. She presented one week postoperatively with a ureterovaginal fistula and required a ureteroneocystostomy after failure of conservative management.

The second complication was in a 74-year-old woman weighing 166 lbs. who had a 1.5-cm cystotomy created during laparoscopic takedown of the bladder. Utilizing our current laparoscopic skills, we would attempt laparoscopic closure of a cystotomy of this nature. However, this was early in our series, and at that time, we had not mastered endoscopic suturing skills. We therefore performed a TAH and BSO through a small Pfannenstiel's incision. This patient was the second who had an abdominal hysterectomy. She was discharged on postoperative day 4.

Our third significant complication occurred in a patient who had congenital right hemidiaphragmatic defects. These defects were discovered high on the dome of the diaphragm during systematic inspection of the intraperitoneal cavity (43). We continued with the procedure, knowing she would probably develop a pneumothorax secondary to the pneumoperitoneum. There were no ventilatory problems during the procedure. Her postoperative chest x-ray, taken in the operating room, revealed a complete right pneumothorax, and a thoracostomy tube was placed. She did well postoperatively and was discharged on hospital day 5.

Three additional patients had minor complications that prolonged their hospital stays. Postoperative ileus was experienced by two patients, ages 71 and 74 years, respectively. Gastric decompression was not required, but oral feedings were delayed. Para-aortic lymphadenectomies for poorly differentiated lesions were performed in each of these patients and both were discharged on postoperative day 5. The third patient developed significant left-sided pulmonary atelectasis postoperatively secondary to intubation of the right mainstem bronchus. This was documented by chest x-ray in the recovery room, obtained because the patient was mildly hypoxic. She did well with aggressive pulmonary toilet but was not discharged until postoperative day 6.

[134]

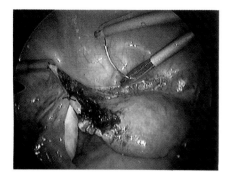

Plate 1 Hemostat grasps tip end of needle as needle holder pulls on suture to turn it to desired orientation.

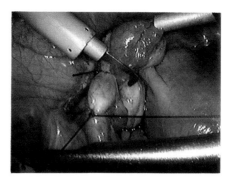

Plate 4 Ligation and division of left infundibulopelvic ligament.

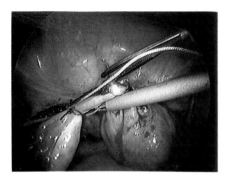

Plate 2 Stitch is completed by grasping tip of needle with hemostat before it is released from needle holder.

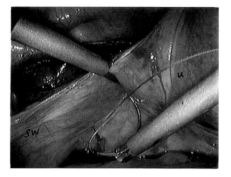

Plate 5 Suture ligation of left uterine artery and upper left cardinal ligament (in grasp of hemostat). U = uterus. SW = pelvic sidewall.

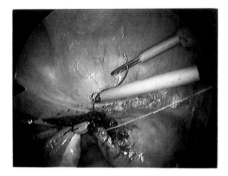

Plate 3 Needle holder grasps suture near needle after it is pulled through tissues by hemostat.

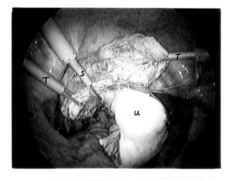

Plate 6 Morcellation of uterine fundus and myomas, using tenaculi to stabilize and spring-retractable scalpel to cut into long narrow strips. U = uterus. T = tenaculum. S = scalpel.

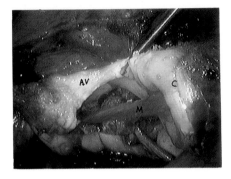

Plate 7 Hemostatic dissection of vagina from cervix with harmonic scalpel. C = cervix. AV = anterior vagina wall. M = cervical mucus.

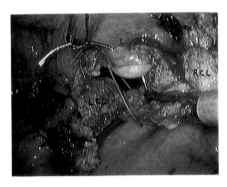

Plate 8 Laparoscopic closure of vagina with interrupted figure-eight stitches. LCL = left cardinal ligament. RCL = right cardinal ligament.

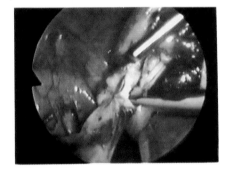

Plate 9 Division of the infundibulopelvic ligament.

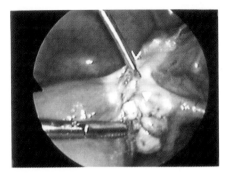

Plate 10 Bladder flap dissection.

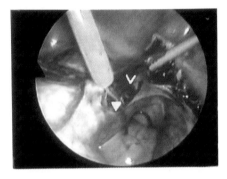

Plate 11 Dissection of the posterior leaf of the broad ligament.

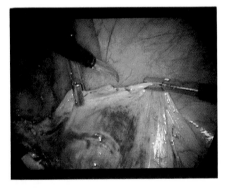

Plate 12 The right round ligament is transected using the scissors as a monopolar electrocautery instrument. Note the traction and countertraction applied by the two grasping instruments.

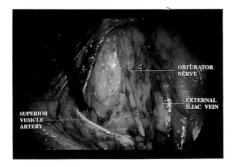

Plate 13 The right broad ligament is opened and a grasper is retracting the right obliterated umbilical ligament (or superior vesical artery), exposing the right obturator nerve and external iliac vein.

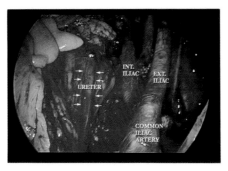

Plate 16 The right medial leaf of the broad ligament is retracted medially, exposing the ureter and the distal common iliac artery. The bifurcation of this artery can be sampled quite adequately laparoscopically.

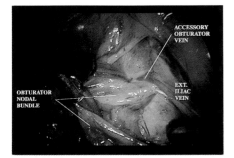

Plate 14 The assistant retracts the right external iliac vein as the surgeon grasps the right obturator nodal bundle and retracts it medially. Scissors are used to separate the nodal bundle from the medial aspect of the external iliac vein. Note an accessory obturator vein traversing through this nodal bundle to empty into the external iliac vein.

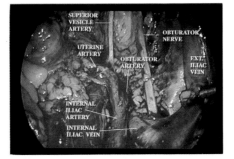

Plate 17 The nodal tissue over the right internal iliac artery and vein and obturator nerve has been removed. Note the origin of the obturator, uterine, and superior vesical arteries.

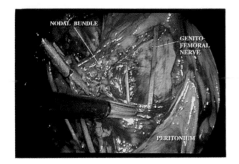

Plate 15 The right external iliac lymph node package is grasped and retracted medially, allowing the surgeon to safely remove the nodes between the genitofemoral nerve and the external iliac vessels.

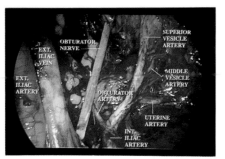

Plate 18 After a left-sided laparoscopic pelvic lymphadenectomy, the external iliac artery and vein, the obturator nerve, and the hypogastric artery can be clearly identified. Note the origin of the obturator, uterine, middle vesical, and superior vesical arteries.

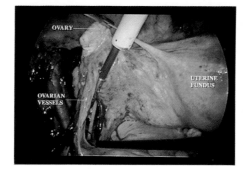

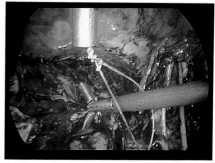

Plate 19 A window has been created in the posterior leaf of the left broad ligament between the uterine vessels and the ureter. This window is extended by blunt dissection.

Plate 22 A grasper placed through the right lateral port is passed through a prefabricated chromic slipknot placed through the suprapubic port prior to grasping the right uterine artery in the area of the lower uterine segment.

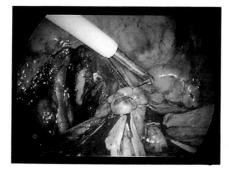

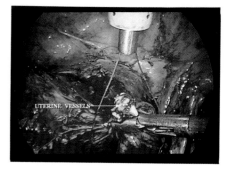

Plate 20 The left infundibulopelvic ligament is ligated extracorporeally using silk suture and the Clarke knot pusher.

Plate 23 After the uterine vessels have been transected, the prefabricated chromic slipknot is passed over these vessels and behind the grasper.

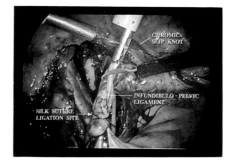

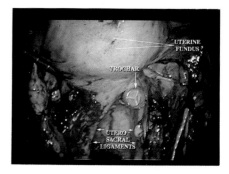

Plate 21 The left infundibulopelvic ligament is being transected with scissors between the grasper and the silk ligation. Note that the grasper has been placed through a prefabricated slipknot inserted through the ipsilateral lateral port.

Plate 24 A disposable trocar without a sleeve has been used to create a colpotomy incision immediately beneath the cervix between the uterosacral ligaments. Once the trocar tip has entered the pelvis, the protective sleeve automatically retracts, covering the tip. Note the blanched appearance of the uterine fundus after ligation of the uterine arteries.

Estimated blood loss in all cases was < 200 cc. There were no other significant short- or long-term complications. The overall average hospital stay was 2.9 days, including the two patients who had pulmonary complications.

Summary

As previously discussed, vaginal hysterectomy has played a limited role in the management of endometrial carcinoma (16–23,25). This approach has, for the most part, been limited because it does not (a) guarantee removal of the adnexa, (b) allow exploration of the intraperitoneal cavity, (c) allow lymph-node sampling, or (d) permit procurement of pelvic washings. In addition, vaginal hysterectomy may not be technically possible in patients with poor descensus and/or pelvic adhesions. In the United States, its use has essentially been limited to medically compromised patients. Indeed, the literature indicates that, in general, vaginal hysterectomy has less morbidity and mortality than abdominal hysterectomy (44–46). The data presented in this series suggest that the morbidity from a LAVH is lower than that of the traditional abdominal staging approach. We believe the one significant complication in this series, a ureteral injury, was completely preventable. Because of our experience and the experiences of others, we believe that for the occasional patient with endometrial cancer in whom the uterine artery cannot be easily ligated vaginally, laparoscopic uterine artery ligation should be accomplished using suture ligation or the bipolar cautery (47). Recent literature also suggests that in addition to lower morbidity and mortality, patients with stage I disease have survival rates with vaginal surgery that are comparable to those of abdominally staged patients (25). Some authors have even suggested a controlled clinical trial comparing abdominal and vaginal hysterectomy in stage I grade 1 or 2 disease (25).

Can laparoscopy detect the metastatic disease that abdominal staging has been shown to discover? Eight of our 61 patients (13%) had metastatic disease, six intraperitoneally and two retroperitoneally. Looked at in another way, metastases were discovered in 35% (8/23) of our patients with grade 2 and 3 lesions. These numbers are consistent with the metastatic rate discovered by abdominal staging (4–11). Metastases to the ovary, peritoneum, omentum, right hemidiaphragm, and pelvic and para-aortic nodes were discovered. We believe an even better evaluation of the peritoneum, especially of the diaphragmatic surfaces, can be obtained laparoscopically because of the magnification offered.

Our overall hospital stay compares favorably to recent studies utilizing an abdominal approach to surgical staging of patients with endometrial cancer. Orr et al. reported a mean hospitalization of six days in 149 patients who were surgically staged (11). Homesley et al., in a retrospective study evaluating the morbidity of selective lymphadenectomy in the surgical staging of endometrial cancer, reported a mean postoperative stay of 10 days for their 281 patients (48). These reports were published in 1991 and 1992, respectively.

[135]

Investigators argue that in performing lymphadenectomy based on tumor grade and depth of invasion, such as our schema, understaging of some patients will occur (11). "Routine" laparoscopic lymphadenectomy could be difficult to accomplish in patients with endometrial cancer since obesity is the most significant limiting factor to this procedure. We were unable to perform the procedure in 6% (2/32) of our patients, and this figure would have undoubtedly been higher if we performed "routine" lymphadenectomy. These obese patients, however, are more likely to have the well-differentiated tumors and, therefore, unlikely to have lymph-node metastases. In our series, the average weight of the 23 patients who did not qualify for lymphadenectomy was 169 lbs., while the average weight of the 32 patients who did or should have had lymphadenectomy according to the schema was 144 lbs. This association between increased weight and well-differentiated lesions has been noted by other authors (49–51). Whether "routine" lymphadenectomy is necessary is debatable because, currently, there are no studies that have documented a survival advantage associated with removal of the lymph nodes.

There are several disadvantages and limitations to the laparoscopic management of patients with early endometrial cancer. First, the laparoscopic surgeon is much more reliant on equipment, operating-room staff, and the surgical assistant than is the surgeon employing laparotomy. Inadequate or malfunctioning equipment, or a staff unfamiliar with laparoscopic troubleshooting, can make even the simplest procedure impossible to perform. Likewise, skills in laparoscopic technique are mandatory for both the surgeon and the assistant during advanced procedures. Since the majority of gynecologic oncologists are not trained in operative laparoscopy, they will be starting at the beginning of a new surgical learning curve, where procedures take longer to perform and the complication rate is higher.

Our experience in oncologic operative laparoscopy verifies the existence of this learning curve. Our initial experiences were difficult and humbling. All of our major complications in this series occurred in the first one third of our patients. However, as experience was gained, complications and operative times decreased. We can currently perform our LASS procedure in about the same time it would take at laparotomy, approximately two hours. We believe that in the future, a significant number of patients with early adenocarcinoma of the endometrium will be managed laparoscopically and vaginally. We suggest that this approach not be used by the "occasional" operative laparoscopist, but be limited to the well-trained, laparoscopically committed gynecologic oncologist.

LASS for stage I endometrial carcinoma is an attractive alternative to the traditional surgical approach. Our initial experience indicates that this approach is feasible, has an acceptable complication rate, and adequately stages these patients. It appears that in the hands of well-trained physicians on properly selected patients, this currently investigational technique may be an important addition to the armamentarium of the gynecologic oncologist.

[136]

References

1 Cullen TH. Cancer of the uterus. Philadelphia: Saunders, 1900.

2 Jones HW. Treatment of adenocarcinoma of the endometrium. Obstet Gynecol Surv 1975;30:147–169.

3 Cheon HK. Prognosis of endometrial carcinoma. Obstet Gynecol 1969;34:680–684.

4 Creasman WT, Boronow RC, Morrow CP, DiSaia PJ, Blessing J. Adenocarcinoma of the endometrium: its metastatic lymph node potential. Gynecol Oncol 1976;4: 239–243.

5 Boronow RC, Morrow CT, Creasman WT, et al. Surgical staging in endometrial cancer: clinical-pathological findings of a prospective study. Obstet Gynecol 1984;63:825–832.

6 Creasman WT, Morrow CP, Bundy BN, Homesley HD, Graham JE, Heller PB. Surgical-pathological spread patterns of endometrial carcinoma: a Gynecologic Oncology Group study. Cancer 1987;60:2035–2041.

7 Lewis BV, Stallworthy JA, Cowdell R. Adenocarcinoma of the body of the uterus. J Obstet Gynaecol Br Common 1970;77:343–348.

8 Musumeci R, DePalo G, Conti U, et al. Are retroperitoneal lymph node metastases a major problem in endometrial carcinoma? Cancer 1980;46:1887–1892.

9 Chen SS. Extrauterine spread in endometrial carcinoma clinically confined to the uterus. Gynecol Oncol 1985;21:23–31.

10 Cowles TA, Magrina JF, Masterson BJ, Capen CV. Comparision of clinical and surgical staging in patients with endometrial carcinoma. Obstet Gynecol 1985; 66:413–416.

11 Orr JW, Holloway RW, Orr PF, Holimon JL. Surgical staging of uterine cancer: an analysis of perioperative morbidity. Gynecol Oncol 1991;12:209–216.

12 Frick HC, Munnell EW, Richart RM, Berger AP, Lawry MF. Carcinoma of the endometrium. Am J Obstet Gynecol 1973;115:663–676.

13 Salazar OM, Bonfiglio TA, Patten SF, et al. Uterine sarcomas: natural history, treatment, and prognosis. Cancer 1978;42:1152–1160.

14 Wharam MD, Phillips TL, Bagshaw MA. The role of radiation therapy in clinical stage I carcinoma of the endometrium. Int J Radiat Oncol Biol Phys 1976;1: 1081–1089.

15 Sheperd JH. Revised FIGO staging for gynecologic cancer. Brit J Obstet Gynaecol 1989;96:889–892.

16 Van Bouwdijk, Bastiaanse MA. Cancer of the body of the uterus. J Obstet Gynaec Br Emp 1952;59:611–616.

17 Ingiulla W, Cosmi EV. Vaginal hysterectomy for the treatment of cancer of the corpus uteri. Am J Obstet Gynecol 1968;100:541–543.

18 Pratt JH. The surgical treatment of cancer of the cervix and uterine fundus. J Florida M A 1954;40:463–470.

19 Pratt JH, Symmonds RE, Welch JS. Vaginal hysterectomy for carcinoma of the fundus. Am J Obstet Gynecol 1964;88:1063–1068.

20 Malkasian GD, McDonald TW, Pratt JH. Carcinoma of the endometrium: Mayo clinical experience. Mayo Clin Proc 1977;52:175–180.

21 Malkasian GD, Annegers JF, Fountain KS. Carcinoma of the endometrium: Stage I. Am J Obstet Gynecol 1980;136:872–883.

22 Candiani GB, Belloni C, Maggi R, Colombo G, Frigoli A, Carinelli SG. Evaluation of different surgical approaches in the treatment of endometrial carcinoma at FIGO stage I. Gynecol Oncol 1990;37:6–8.

23 Peters WA, Andersen WA, Thornton N, Morley GW. The selective use of vaginal hysterectomy in the management of adenocarcinoma of the endometrium. Am J Obstet Gynecol 1983;146:285–291.

24 Lurain JR. The significance of positive peritoneal cytology in endometrial carcinoma. Gynecol Oncol 1992;46:143–144.

25 Bloss JD, Berman ML, Bloss LP, Buller RE. Use of vaginal hysterectomy for the management of stage I endometrial carcinoma in the medically compromised patient. Gynecol Oncol 1991;40:74–77.

26 Reich H, DeCaprio J, McGlynn F. Laparoscopic hysterectomy. J Gynecol Surg 1989;5:213–215.

27 Mage G, Canis M, Wittiez A, Pouly MA, Bruhat MA. Hysterectomie et coelioscopie. J Gynecol Oncol Biol Reprod 1990;19:569–573.

28 Minelli L, Angiolillo M, Caione C, Palmer V. Laparoscopically assisted vaginal hysterectomy. Endoscopy 1991;23:64–66.

29 Liu CY. Laparoscopic hysterectomy: a review of 72 cases. J Reprod Med 1992; 37:351–354.

30 Summit RL Jr, Stovall TG, Lipscomb GH, Ling FW. Randomized comparision of laparoscopic-assisted vaginal hysterectomy with standard vaginal hysterectomy in an outpatient setting. Obstet Gynecol 1992;80:895–901.

31 Padial JG, Sotolongo J, Casey MJ, Johnson C, Osborne NG. Laparoscopy-assisted vaginal hysterectomy: report of seventy-five consecutive cases. J Gynecol Surg 1992;8:81–85.

32 Wurtz A, Mazeman E, Gosselin B, Woelffle D, Sauvage L, Rousseau O. Bilan anatomique des adénopathies rétropéritonéales par endoscopie chirurgicale. Ann Chir 1987;41:258–263.

33 Dargent D, Salvat J. L'Envahissement ganglionnaire pelvien. Paris: MEDSI, Mc-Graw Hill, 1989.

34 Querleu D, Leblanc E, Castelain B. Laparoscopic pelvic lymphadenectomy in the staging of early carcinoma of the cervix. Am J Obstet Gynecol 1991;164:579–581.

35 Childers JM, Surwit EA. Laparoscopic para-aortic lymph node biopsy for diagnosis of a non-Hodgkin's lymphoma. Surg Laparosc Endoscop 1992;2:139–142.

36 Childers JM, Surwit EA. Combined laparoscopic and vaginal surgery for the management of two cases of stage I endometrial cancer. Gynecol Oncol 1992;45:46–51.

37 American College of Obstetricians and Gynecologists. Gynecologic Oncology Group surgical procedures manual. Washington: American College of Obstetricians and Gynecologists, 1989;48.

38 Childers JM, Hatch KD, Tran AN, Surwit EA. Laparoscopic para-aortic lymphadenectomy in gynecologic malignancies. Obstet Gynecol 1993;82:741–747.

39 Childers JM, Brzechffa PR, Surwit EA. Laparoscopy using the left upper quandrant as the primary trocar site. Gynecol Oncol 1993;50:221–225.

40 Herd J, Fowler J, Shenson D, Lacy S, Montz F. Laparoscopic para-aortic lymph node sampling: development of a technique. Gyn Oncol 1992;44:271–276.

41 Spirtos NM, Schlaerth JB, Indman PD, et al. Laparoscopic bilateral pelvic and aortic lymph node sampling: a new technique. Poster presentation, American College of Obstetricians and Gynecologists, May 4, 1993, Washington, D.C.

42 Childers JM, Huang D, Surwit EA. Laparoscopic trocar-assisted colpotomy. Obstet Gynecol 1993;81:153–155.

43 Childers JM, Caplinger P. Spontaneous pneumothorax during operative laparoscopy secondary to congenital diaphragmatic defects. J Reprod Med 1993, in press.

44 Pitkin RM. Abdominal hysterectomy in obese women. Surg Gynecol Obstet 1976; 142:532–536.

45 Pitkin RM. Vaginal hysterectomy in obese women. Obstet Gynecol 1977;49:567–569.

46 Wingo PA, Huezo CM, Rubin GL, Ory HW, Peterson HB. The mortality risk associated with hysterectomy. Am J Obstet Gynecol 1985;152:803–808.

47 Woodland MB. Ureteral injury during laparoscopy-assisted vaginal hysterectomy with the endoscopic linear stapler. Am J Obstet Gynecol 1992;167:756–757.

48 Homesley HD, Kadar N, Barrett RJ, Lentz SS. Selective pelvic and para-aortic lymphadenectomy does not increase morbidity in surgical staging of endometrial cancer. Am J Obstet Gynecol 1992;167:1225–1230.

49 Cauppila A, Grönroos M, Nieminen U. Clinical outcome in endometrial cancer. Obstet Gynecol 1982;60:473–480.

50 Bokhman JV. Two pathogenic types of endometrial carcinoma. Gynecol Oncol 1983;15:10–17.

51 Larson DM, Johnson K, Olson KA. Pelvic and para-aortic lymphadenectomy for surgical staging of endometrial cancer: morbidity and mortality. Obstet Gynecol 1992;79:998–1001.

11 Abdominal Myomectomy

EUGENE F. GUERRE, JR.

Leiomyomata are the most common solid tumors of the female pelvis and are responsible for one third of hospital admissions to gynecologic services (1). Ranney (2) reported that in 55% of 1022 surgical patients, myomas were a major indication. It also appears that leiomyomata occur three to nine times more frequently in the Afro-American population than in the Caucasian.

It is well known that the growth of leiomyomata is estrogen-dependent; however, both estrogen and progesterone receptors have been found in leiomyomata. A current debate questions whether the estrogen concentration in myomas is the same as in normal myometrium. Soules et al. (3) demonstrated a cyclic rise and fall in the number of receptors similar to that seen in normal myometrium. Whereas Wilson et al. (4) showed an increase in the number of estrogen receptors in leiomyomas, Pollow et al. (5) and Puuka et al. (6), in separate studies, demonstrated normal concentrations of estrogen and progesterone receptors.

Clinical aspects of uterine leiomyomata

The vast majority of uterine leiomyomata are asymptomatic and best left alone, particularly since the rate of sarcomatous degeneration is so low. Novak (7), in 1958, reported an incidence of 0.7%. A review by Montague et al. (8) in 1965 of 13,000 myomas resulted in an incidence of 0.29%. An even lower incidence was reported by Conscaden and Singh (9) of 0.04%–0.13%. The true incidence is probably around 0.1% or one in 1000. Rapid growth, however, particularly in the older female, would warrant its removal.

On the other hand, it is estimated that 20–50% of women with myomas will be symptomatic. Symptoms include abnormal bleeding, pelvic pain or pressure, or impingement on surrounding structures. Menorrhagia is the symptom most frequently reported in association with leiomyomata. Several explanations for this have been proposed. Submucous myomas are frequently associated with abnormal bleeding, possibly secondary to ulcerations on the tumor. However, since only 5% of all myomas are submucous, this does not completely explain the high incidence of menorrhagia. Other theories include an association with anovulation (10), larger endometrial surface area in uteri with myomas

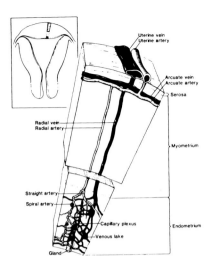

Figure 11-1 Normal uterus. (Copyright Baylor College of Medicine, 1980, P. Smith. From Buttram VC, Reiter RC. Surgical treatment of the infertile female. 1985. Reprinted with permission from Williams and Wilkins, Baltimore, Maryland.)

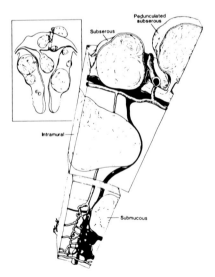

Figure 11-2 Myomatous uterus. (Copyright Baylor College of Medicine, 1980, P. Smith. From Buttram VC, Reiter RC. Surgical treatment of the infertile female. 1985. Reprinted with permission from Williams and Wilkins, Baltimore, Maryland.)

(11), and interference with normal uterine contractibility (12). None of these have been adequately substantiated.

Perhaps the most intriguing theory for internal bleeding in patients with leiomyomas was developed by Farrer-Brown et al. (13). They have proposed that myomas impinge and compress the veins of the inner myometrium resulting in venous congestion and dilation of the adjacent endometrial venous plexus (Figures 11-1 and 11-2).

Approximately one third of patients with leiomyomas will complain of pelvic pain or pressure, two frequent indicators for surgery. The cause of the pain is unclear and may be due to secondary pelvic conditions, such as adenomyosis, endometriosis, or pelvic adhesions. Pelvic pressure is a common complaint in patients with large myomas, most commonly involving the bladder, resulting in urinary frequency, retention, or overflow incontinence.

There is a significantly increased rate of spontaneous abortion in patients with leiomyomata. In a review by Buttram and Reiter (14) in 1981, there was a 41% incidence of spontaneous abortion prior to myomectomy. This rate was reduced to 19% after myomectomy. Several mechanisms have been proposed to explain the increased rate of pregnancy loss. These include increased uterine instability and contractibility, disturbances in uterine blood flow and blood supply to the endometrium, enlargement of the uterine cavity, and thin, poorly vascularized endometrium overlying submucous myomas.

Less clear is the association of uterine leiomyomata with infertility. Buttrum and Reiter (15) studied 1,698 cases of myomectomy, but found only 27% infertile. This study suggests that these tumors do not significantly contribute to the overall incidence of fertility. Obvious explanations for their adverse effects on fertility include impingement on the interstitial portions of the fallopian tubes, enlargement and distortion of the endometrial cavity, particularly by submucous myomas, and impingement on the endocervical canal. Other less clear explanations include an association with anovulation (10), increased myometrial irritation and hypercontractibility (16), and altered interuterine blood flow and resulting menorrhagia (13,17).

Minimizing blood loss

Since myomectomy can result in considerable blood loss, hemostasis at the time of surgery becomes a major consideration. Several methods to control blood loss are available. Bonney (18) designed a clamp to compress the uterine arteries as well as to help stabilize the uterus. Lock (19) recommended using rubber-shod sponge forceps for occlusion of the uterine and ovarian arteries. Rubin (20) used a rubber catheter by passing it through small incisions made beneath the round ligaments and encircling it around the lower uterine segment to occlude the uterine vessels. These authors recommend releasing the compression about every 10–20 minutes to prevent possible ischemic necrosis to the myometrium as well as to prevent the potential building of histamine-like substances in the uterus.

[140]

Injection of diluted vasopressin (20u/100 cc solution) is popular for reducing perioperative bleeding. The solution is injected at the junction of the myoma with the myometrium as well as at the base of the myoma. The effect lasts for approximately 30 minutes and it does not mask arterial bleeding. Dillon (21) found that with the administration of vasopressin, 72% of patients did not require blood replacement, whereas only 43% of controls did not require replacement. These results were reaffirmed by Ingersoll and Malone (22).

Although the above-described techniques can help reduce intraoperative blood loss, there is no substitute for careful, meticulous surgical technique with particular attention to bleeding vessels as they are encountered. Gentle traction on the tumor as it is dissected from its pseudocapsule is emphasized. Vigorous pulling and twisting will tear blood vessels and result in more bleeding. Blunt finger dissection should be avoided in favor of sharp dissection to minimize excessive bleeding and avoid unnecessary entry into the endometrial cavity. Care needs to be exercised when dissecting laterally to avoid bleeding into the broad ligament.

In recent years, the availability of autologous blood transfusion, pharmacologic agents such as GnRH agonist, and controlled hypotensive anesthesia have further reduced the risk of bleeding during myomectomy.

GnRH agonists are useful preoperatively to help correct anemic states, which are frequently encountered in symptomatic patients with a history of menorrhagia, and to help decrease intraoperative blood loss. Friedman (23) demonstrated significant increases with hemoglobin, hematocrit, serum Fe, and total iron-binding capacity in patients treated with 8–24 weeks of GnRH agonist.

Stovall et al. (24) were able to demonstrate significant reduction in intraoperative blood loss after two months of treatment with GnRH agonist. Friedman et al. (25) also found significant reduction in intraoperative blood loss compared with controls in patients with uterine volumes greater than 600 cm³, but no difference was found with small (<600 cm³) uterine volume.

Therefore, it appears that GnRH agonist should be given serious consideration for preoperative use in patients who present with significant anemia or those with large myomatous uteri.

With the risk of acquiring infectious diseases such as AIDS through homologous blood transfusion, there has been a rapidly growing interest in autologous blood transfusions by patients prior to surgery, even though the risk of acquiring HIV from a transfusion is very small (1:400,000 to 1:1,000,000) (26). In general, the patient should have a hematocrit of at least 34%, and may donate one unit per week. The last unit is collected no sooner than 72 hours prior to surgery. Iron supplementation is prescribed during this period. It is usually recommended that the patient have two units of blood available prior to surgery.

Another method to reduce the need for homologous blood transfusion in patients with significant intraoperative blood loss during myomec-

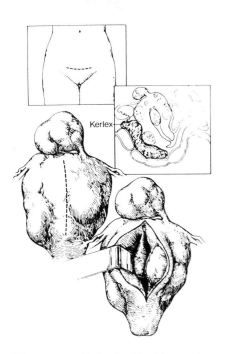

Figure 11-3 Abdominal incision and anterior midline vertical incision. (Copyright Baylor College of Medicine, 1980, P. Smith. From Buttram VC, Reiter RC. Surgical treatment of the infertile female. 1985. Reprinted with permission from Williams and Wilkins, Baltimore, Maryland.)

Figure 11-4 Diagrammatic representation of the uterine anatomy. Radial arteries branch in the inner third of the myometrium into straight and coiled (spiral) arteries. The straight arteries pass as far as the basal endometrium, and the spiral arteries follow a coiled course through the endometrium. (From Hunt RB. Atlas of female infertility surgery. Second edition. 1992. Reprinted with permission from Mosby Yearbook, Inc., St. Louis, Missouri.)

tomy is intraoperative autotransfusion. This procedure is made possible with the use of the Cell Saver (Haemonetics Corporation, Braintree, MA). Blood is suctioned from the operative field, autocoagulated, filtered, packed, washed in saline, then concentrated. The blood is then infused back into the patient. Because the procedure is rather costly, it is probably only useful in patients with blood losses greater than 1000 cc.

Controlled hypotensive anesthesia has been shown to be useful in reducing intraoperative bleeding. By using vasodilating agents, such as nitroglycerin, epidural or spinal anesthesia, or selected inhalational agents, one can reduce venous tone and maintain a mean blood pressure of 60 mmHg. In 1983, Powell et al. (27) reported a 70% decrease in blood loss in 26 patients undergoing radical hysterectomy and lymphadenectomy. Only 11.5% of those in whom controlled hypotensive anesthesia was used required transfusion compared to 81% in the control group.

Technique of abdominal myomectomy

For uteri 10–12 weeks in size or less, a transverse incision is generally adequate. However, if the uterus is greater than 12 weeks in size, a vertical incision is preferred. Adequate exposure is of utmost importance. A self-retaining retractor is quite useful for maintaining exposure and enables the surgical assistant to perform other tasks, such as suctioning and irrigation. Suction is preferred to using sponges to remove blood and irrigant from the operative field. Laparotomy packs can be placed in sterile plastic bags or talc-free gloves prior to using them for packing the bowel. They may also be placed in the cul-de-sac to elevate the uterus.

A single vertical midline uterine incision is optimal for two reasons (Figure 11-3). Anterior incisions are less likely to result in adhesion formation than posterior incisions, and midline incisions will result in less bleeding than more lateral incisions because blood supply to the uterus is by horizontal concentric loops (Figure 11-4). If anterior adhesions do form, they are less likely to involve the adnexa. Tumors more

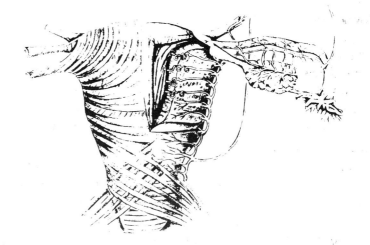

[142]

lateral to the midline incision can be removed through this incision by making secondary myometrial incisions and pushing the myomas medially toward the primary incision (Figure 11-5). This primary anterior incision can be extended toward the cervix to remove anterior cervical myomas after developing and reflecting the bladder flap or toward the fundus as necessary.

Posterior incisions are associated with a high risk of adhesion formation with involvement of the adnexa. Therefore, if at all possible, posterior myomas are best removed through a fundal extension of the anterior incision. If the endometrial cavity has already been opened to remove submucous myomas, one may remove posterior tumors through the endometrial cavity and anterior uterine incision, as advocated by Bonney (18) (Figure 11-6). However, because of the risk of development of intrauterine synechiae, it cannot be recommended routinely for removing all posterior myomas. Instead, to avoid endometrial cavity damage, it is best to make a midline posterior uterine incision to remove posterior myomas.

The enlarging fibroid places pressure on the surrounding myometrium. This thinned myometrium, or pesudocapsule, encapsulates the myomas, providing a well-defined cleavage plane between the fibroid and its pseudocapsule. To minimize blood loss, it is extremely important to identify this plane. Many times, the surgeon will dissect outside this plane within a well-vascularized myometrium with resultant increased blood loss. Dissection along the pseudocapsule is best accomplished by meticulous sharp dissection with Metzenbaum scissors. Vigorous blunt dissection using one's finger may result in increased bleeding. A tenaculum or towel clip is useful for maintaining traction on the myoma. A Kelly clamp is placed on the pedicle at the base of the myoma, allowing the placement of a suture ligature for hemostasis. This technique is preferable to blindly placing sutures at the base of the defect in an attempt to control bleeding.

If the endometrial cavity has been opened, the edges should be carefully approximated with 3-0 or 4-0 absorbable suture, such as Dexon or Vicryl. The uterine defect is generally closed in two layers. A purse-string suture or figure-eight suture using 2-0 Dexon or Vicryl is used to close the myometrium, eliminate dead space, and establish hemostasis. Placement of this first layer of sutures needs to extend to the base of the myometrial incision to prevent hematoma formation. Suture placement adjacent to the interstitial portion of the fallopian tube needs to be done very meticulously to avoid inadvertent occlusion of the oviduct. Excess myometrium and serosa may be excised. After the full thickness of the incision has been closed, the serosa may be approximated and closed using a subserosal or running suture of 3-0 or 4-0 Vicryl or Dexon (Figure 11-7).

Adhesion prevention

The formation of adhesions following myomectomy is always of concern, particularly if there is a posterior incision. Several methods for prevention of adhesions may be considered. During the procedure, use

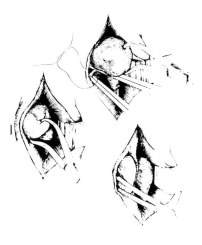

Figure 11-5 Enucleation of intramural leiomyoma. (Copyright Baylor College, 1980, P. Smith. From Buttram VC, Reiter RC. Surgical treatment of the infertile female. 1985. Reprinted with permission from Williams and Wilkins, Baltimore, Maryland.)

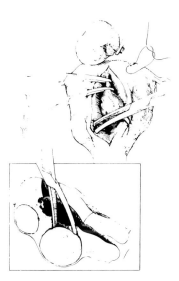

Figure 11-6 Removal of subserous, intramural submucous tumors and transcavitary enucleation (Copyright Baylor College, 1980, P. Smith. From Buttram VC, Reiter RC. Surgical treatment of the infertile female. 1985. Reprinted with permission from Williams and Wilkins, Baltimore, Maryland.)

[143]

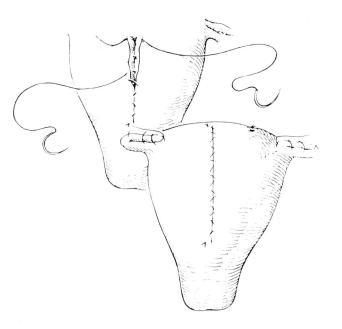

Figure 11-7 Closure of uterine incision. (Copyright Baylor College, 1980, P. Smith. From Buttram VC, Reiter RC. Surgical treatment of the infertile female. 1985. Reprinted with permission from Williams and Wilkins, Baltimore, Maryland.)

of heparinized irrigation may reduce fibrin formation, which leads to adhesion formation. Typically, 5000 U of heparin is placed in 1 L of Ringer's lactate for this purpose.

Exposed laparotomy packs, even when moist, can scratch the peritoneal surface, resulting in adhesion formation. An alternative is to place the packs in either sterile plastic bags or talc-free gloves prior to placement in the abdomen or pelvis.

Barriers may be considered to cover the uterine incision(s), particularly the posterior ones. One alternative is Interceed TC-7, which is composed of oxidized regenerated cellulose. The operative site, however, has to be completely dry and blood-free prior to placement. The presence of blood at the site may actually contribute to increased adhesion formation. Another alternative is the use of Gore-Tex surgical membrane, a nonreactive expanded polytetrafluoroethylene. Boyers et al. (28) showed a significant reduction in adhesion formation in the pelvic sidewall and uterine horn on New Zealand rabbits. The Gore-Tex is held in place by suturing each corner to the uterine serosa with a 5-0 nonabsorbable suture. Absorbable suture should be avoided; otherwise, the Gore-Tex may become free-floating within the pelvis and abdomen.

For those with a posterior incision or a retroflexed or retroverted uterus, one may consider a uterine suspension. A simple method of suspension is triplication of the round ligaments using 3-0 nylon suture. This usually results in adequate elevation of the body of the uterus out of the cul-de-sac.

Management guidelines for leiomyomata

The patient's desire for future childbearing is the greatest reason for contemplating a myomectomy. Unless the uterus is very large or symptomatic, she may consider pregnancy now since myomectomy itself can result in formation of pelvic adhesions and reduced fertility, as suggested by Berkeley et al. (29) Therefore, the benefits of myomectomy must clearly outweigh its risk.

Seldom is infertility the single indication for myomectomy. In fact, it is extremely important to perform a complete evaluation of the infertile couple. Frequently, other factors will be uncovered, such as tubal obstruction or pelvic adhesions. On the other hand, if a hystersalpingogram shows obstruction of the interstitial portion of a fallopian tube, or enlargement and distortion of the uterine cavity, myomectomy is justified.

Does myomectomy improve pregnancy rates? This problem was addressed by Babaknia et al. (30) at Johns Hopkins in 1978. They reported on 34 patients with primary infertility and 12 with secondary infertility. All patients had no other explanations for their infertility. After myomectomy, 38% of the patients with primary infertility conceived and 50% of the patients with secondary infertility conceived. Of 75 patients treated with myomectomy for infertility by Ingersoll and Malone (22), one half became pregnant within two years or surgery. In 1993, Berkeley et al. (29) reviewed the results of fifty myomectomies. Although there were 36 subsequent pregnancies, only 16% of infertile couples with an otherwise completely normal evaluation conceived, suggesting that myomectomy may not be justified in couples with normal evaluations.

In a review of the medical literature, including their own data, Buttrum and Reiter (14) studied 285 patients with leiomyoma and menorrhagia who underwent myomectomy. Eighty-one percent had resolution of menorrhagia. Of the 76 infertile couples in whom a myomatous uterus was the only abnormality, 54% conceived after myomectomy.

Figure 11-8 provides an outline for management of patients with leiomyomata. Patients with small uteri, less than 10–12 weeks, who are asymptomatic without any growth may be observed until pregnancy is desired. Similarly, a trial of conception is warranted in this population if the patient is desirous of pregnancy now. Patients with uteri larger than 12 weeks in size or with evidence of continued growth who desire pregnancy now or in the future would benefit from myomectomy. Hysterectomy is indicated in the symptomatic patient who does not desire future fertility. Finally, patients with leiomyomas who desire pregnancy now or later who are symptomatic (abnormal bleeding, recurrent abortion,

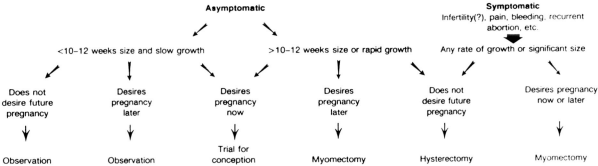

Figure 11-8 Management of nonpregnant patients with uterine leiomyomata. (From Leiomyomata uteri and abdominal hysterectomy for benign disease. In: Mattingly RF, Thompson JD, eds. TeLinde's operative gynecology. 6th edition. Philadelphia: J.B. Lippincott Co., 1985. Reproduced with permission of the publisher, J.B. Lippincott Co.)

rapid growth) or those in whom infertility is the result of proximal occlusion of the fallopian tubes or an abnormal or enlarged endometrial cavity would benefit from myomectomy.

In discussing myomectomy with the patient, the risk of recurrence should be addressed. Brown et al. (31) followed 176 patients for five years after myomectomy and found 31.3% had recurrence of leiomyoma. Hysterectomy was performed in 16.5%. Malone (16) found that if myomectomy was done in patients with solitary tumors, subsequent hysterectomy rate was 11% versus 26% in patients with multiple myomas.

Summary

Uterine leiomyomata are the most common solid tumors of the female pelvis and are frequently encountered by the gynecologist. Generally, small asymptomatic myomas may be simply observed. Myomectomy should be considered in symptomatic patients or those who have larger or growing tumors and desire preservation of fertility. Patients not desirous of maintaining their fertility may choose hysterectomy. However, especially today, this is not always the case. There is a growing demand for uterine preservation in today's female population. Many women feel that preservation of the uterus and menstrual function is essential to health, youth, and sexual life. In-depth discussion with the patient is extremely important, including risk/benefit ratios of hysterectomy versus myomectomy. Recurrence rate of myomas after myomectomy should also be addressed, and, of course, the patient needs to be informed of the small risk that the uterus may need to be removed if bleeding becomes a serious problem at the time of myomectomy.

Methods of reducing the risk of hemorrhage have been discussed, including the use of dilute vasopressin, midline uterine incision, tourniquets, autologous blood transfusion, and hypotensive anesthesia. Adequate exposure and meticulous dissection with special attention to bleeders cannot be over-emphasized.

Postoperative adhesion formation may be minimized by use of heparinized irrigants, placing laparotomy sponges in plastic bags or talc-free gloves, minimizing the amount of clotted blood in the operative field by gentle suction (not sponges), and covering the uterine incision with Interceed TC-7 or, preferably, Gore-Tex surgical membrane.

Finally, a plan of management for patients with uterine fibroids has been presented. Hopefully, by following the guidelines presented in this chapter, an optimal outcome can be achieved during and following abdominal myomectomy.

References

1 Baggish MS. Mesenchymal tumors of the uterus. Clin Obstet Gynecol 1974;17:51.
2 Ranney B, Frederick I. The occasional need for myomectomy. Obstet Gynecol 1979;53:437.
3 Soules MR, McCarty KS. Leiomyomas: steroid receptor contents. Am J Obstet Gynecol 1982;143:6.

[146]

4 Wilson EA, Yang F, Rees ED. Estradiol and progesterone binding in uterine leiomyomata and in normal uterine tissue. Obstet Gynecol 1980;55:20.

5 Pollow K, Guilfuss J, Boquoi E, Pollow B. Estrogen and progesterone binding proteins in normal human myometrium and leiomyoma tissue. J Clin Chem Biochem 1978;16:503.

6 Puuka MJ, Kontula KK, Kouppila AJI, Janne OA, Vihko RK. Estrogen receptor in human myoma tissue. Mol Cell Endocrinol 1976;6:35.

7 Novak ER. Benign and malignant changes in uterine myomas. Clin Obstet Gynecol 1958;1:421.

8 Montague A, Schwartz DP, Woodruff JD. Sarcoma arising in leiomyoma of uterus: factors influencing prognosis. Am J Obstet Gynecol 1965;92:421.

9 Corscaden JA, Sinjh BP. Leiomyosarcoma of the uterus. Am J Obstet Gynecol 1958;75:149.

10 Miller NF, Ludovici PP. On the origin and development of uterine fibroids. Am J Obstet Gynecol 1955;70:720.

11 Sehgal N, Haskins AL. The mechanism of uterine bleeding in the presence of fibromyomas. Am J Surg 1960;26:21.

12 Faulkner RL. The blood vessels of the myomatous uterus. Am J Obstet Gynecol 1944;47:185.

13 Farrer-Brown G, Bailby JOW, Tarbit MH. Venous changes in the endometrium of the myomatous uterus. Obstet Gynecol 1971;38:743.

14 Buttram VC, Reiter RC. Uterine leiomyomata: etiology, symptomatology, and management. Fertil Steril 1981;36:433.

15 Buttram VC, Reiter RC. Uterine leiomyomata. In: Carol Lynn Brown, ed. Surgical treatment of the infertile patient. Baltimore: Williams and Wilkins, 1985:204–205.

16 Malone LJ, Ingersoll FM. Myomectomy in infertility. In: Behaman SJ, Kistner RW, eds. Progress in infertility. Vol 2. Boston: Little Brown, 1975:85.

17 Farrer-Brown G, Beilby JOW, Tarbit MH. The vascular patterns in myomatous uteri. J Obstet Gynaecol Br Commonw 1970;77:967.

18 Bonney V. The technique and results of myomectomy. Lancet 1931;220:171.

19 Lock FR. Multiple myomectomy. Am J Obstet Gynecol 1969:104:642.

20 Rubin IC. Uterine fibromyomas and sterility. Clin Obstet Gynecol 1958;1:501.

21 Dillon TF. Control of blood loss during gynecologic surgery. Obstet Gynecol 1962;19:428.

22 Ingersoll FM, Malone LJ. Myomectomy: an alternative to hysterectomy. Arch Surg 1970;100:557.

23 Friedman AJ, Barbieri RL, Doubilet PM, et al. A radmonized, double-blind trial of gonadotropin-releasing hormone agonist (leuprolide) with or without medroxyprogesterone acetate in the treatment of leiomyomata uteri. Fertil Steril 1988;49:404–409.

24 Stovall TG, Ling FW, Henry LC, Woodruff MR. A randomized trial evaluating leuprolide acetate before hysterectomy as treatment for leiomyomas. Am J Obstet Gynecol 1991;164:1420–1425.

25 Friedman AJ, Rein MS, Harrison-Atlas D, et al. A randomized, placebo-controlled, double blind study evaluating leuprolide acetate depot treatment before myomectomy. Fertil Steril 1989;52:728–733.

26 Axelrod FB, Pepkowitz SH, Goldfinger D. Establishment of a schedule of optimal preoperative collection of autologous blood. Obstet Gynecol Surv 1990;45:331–333.

27 Powell JL, Mogelnichi SR, Franklin EW, et al. A deliberate hypotensive technique for decreasing blood loss during radical hysterectomy and pelvic lymphadenectomy. Am J Obstet Gyncol 1983;147:196–202.

28 Boyers SP, Diamond MP, DeCherney AH. Reduction in postoperative adhesions in the rabbit with Gore-Tex surgical membrane. Fertil Steril 1988;49:1066.

29 Berkeley AS, DeCherney AH, Polan ML. Abdominal myomectomy and subsequent fertility. Surg Gynecol Obstet 1983;156:319.

30 Babaknia A, Rock RA, Jones HW. Pregnancy success following abdominal myomectomy for infertility. Fertil Steril 1978;30:644.

31 Brown JM, Malkasian GD, Symmonds RE. Abdominal myomectomy. Am J Obstet Gynecol 1967;99:126.

12 Laparoscopic Myomectomy

LARRY DEAN GURLEY

Leiomyomata uteri, the most common tumors of the female pelvis, occur in 25% to 50% of women and are estimated to be responsible for approximately one third of hospital admissions to gynecology services (1,2). Many patients with symptomatic uterine fibroids desire conservation of the uterus to allow attempts at future conception or in order to avoid hysterectomy. There is a renewed interest in abdominal myomectomy in the reproductive age patient (3,4). The reader is referred to The American Fertility Society's *Guideline for Practice: Myomas and Reproductive Dysfunction,* published in 1992, for an excellent review of the implications of uterine fibroids in the reproductive age woman.

Operative laparoscopy is increasingly replacing laparotomy for the treatment of numerous gynecological problems. Several authors have reported their experience with laparoscopic removal of symptomatic uterine fibroids (5,6,7). In 1994, myomectomy by laparotomy remains the standard of care for patients with symptomatic uterine fibroids who desire future childbearing.

Indications for laparoscopic myomectomy

Patients selected as candidates for laparoscopic myomectomy should have symptoms attributed to uterine fibroids which are not relieved by conservative methods, including the use of nonsteroidal anti-inflammatory drugs or low dose oral contraceptives. Patients in the perimenopausal age group may benefit from short-term treatment with GnRH agonists with the expectation that symptoms from their uterine fibroids will regress as they enter menopause. The presence of pelvic endometriosis can confound the diagnosis of dysmenorrhea or pelvic pain secondary to uterine fibroids and must be considered.

Contraindications to laparoscopic myomectomy

Infertile patients who desire immediate conception should undergo a complete infertility evaluation and an appropriate trial of conception prior to consideration of myomectomy (8). As there is no long-term follow-up yet available to assess the risk of uterine dehiscence during pregnancies following laparoscopic myomectomy, and a recent case report describes this complication (9), desire for future childbearing

[148]

should be considered a relative contraindication for laparoscopic myomectomy in cases of intramural fibroids. Lack of the surgeon's ability to suture laparoscopically precludes any attempt at myomectomy except in the case of extremely superficial subserosal or pedunculated fibroids. Myoma size over 10 cm is a relative contraindication because of the excessive time required for removal of the tumor from the peritoneal cavity using currently available morcellation devices and techniques.

The surgeon should make a decision at the time of the myomectomy concerning recommendation for the route of delivery during subsequent pregnancies. Cesarean section is generally recommended if the endometrium has been incised or if the myometrial dissection is extensive (1). Until more information is gathered concerning laparoscopic myomectomy, the author recommends cesarean section as the mode of delivery in any patient who has undergone laparoscopic removal of an intramural fibroid.

Leiomyosarcoma may be difficult to diagnose preoperatively (10). Suspicion of leiomyosarcoma and treatment by laparotomy should be undertaken in any reproductive aged patient with rapid growth of uterine fibroids or with documented growth of uterine fibroids in a postmenopausal patient.

Preparation of the patient

Informed consent

Consent is obtained, discussing fully the risks of infection, hemorrhage, transfusion with related risks, injury to internal organs, and need for laparotomy. Patients who elect this procedure and desire future childbearing are counseled that delivery by cesarean section will be recommended unless the fibroid removed is purely subserosal. Patients are made aware that in 30% of cases, myoma recurrence will follow myomectomy (8). Hysterectomy is offered as definitive therapy to those patients not desiring future childbearing.

Preoperative care

Patients with previous episodes of abnormal uterine bleeding should undergo endometrial sampling prior to admission to rule out endometrial hyperplasia or carcinoma. The presumed number and location of fibroids should be determined by preoperative pelvic ultrasound examination, which also rules out any ovarian process. The patient is admitted on the morning of surgery and is given a single dose of a first-generation cephalosporin.

Pretreatment of patients for two to three months with leuprolide acetate depot has been shown to lead to reduction in intraoperative blood loss during abdominal myomectomy in women with large uterine fibroids (11). It has been shown that an increased risk of fibroid recurrence is not associated with preoperative use of leuprolide acetate but is associated with removal of four or more fibroids (12). It is this author's experience, however, that pretreatment with leuprolide acetate depot may make the distinction between myoma capsule and myometrium more difficult to determine, with resultant difficulty in developing surgical planes. Currently, the author uses leuprolide acetate depot only to pretreat patient's with fibroids over 6 cm in size.

Technique for laparoscopic myomectomy

The patient is placed in the dorsal low lithotomy position. The thighs should be only slightly flexed to allow full motion of instruments in the suprapubic and low lateral operating ports. If not performed previously, a hysteroscopic exam is carried out to evaluate the endometrial cavity for submucosal fibroids. Diagnostic laparoscopy is then carried out in standard fashion with a 10-mm port in the umbilical incision through which the telescope and a midline suprapubic trocar sleeve for manipulation of the pelvic organs are placed. It is important at this time to evaluate the uterine landmarks, specifically the round ligaments and tubes bilaterally, to accurately determine the position of the uterine fibroids. Occasionally, a fibroid will appear remarkably like the uterine fundus. Accurate localization of the uterine fundus is necessary to ensure correct placement of the uterine incision for the myomectomy.

At this time, the surgeon will determine whether or not a laparoscopic approach is reasonable. This decision will be based on the surgeon's experience, the number of myomas, and the position of the myomas. If a decision is made to proceed with laparoscopic myomectomy, two more 5-mm trocars are placed in the Pfannenstiel line, one trocar lateral to each set of inferior epigastric vessels. Inferior epigastric vessels, arising from the external iliac artery in the region of the internal inguinal ring, are visualized using the laparoscope. The vessels are lateral to the obliterated umbilical ligament and are visible in most patients.

The initially placed 5-mm suprapubic trocar may be changed during the course of the surgery for a 12-mm trocar, or a minilaparotomy incision may be made in this area for extraction of the fibroid mass.

Using a 20-gauge spinal needle connected to a 10-cc syringe with an IV extension tubing, a solution of 5 units of vasopressin (Pitressin, Parke-Davis, Morris Plains, NJ) in 100 cc of normal saline is used for vasoconstriction. Ten to 30 cc of this solution are injected around the base of the fibroid(s). The uterine serosa is then opened with hook scissors, taking care to direct the incision so that it may be extended, if needed, without entering the lateral lower uterine segment or the cornual region. Alternately, unipolar cautery or laser energy may be used for the uterine incision and to aid during subsequent dissection. Several steps may be required during this initial incision to make sure the correct plane has been reached. If there is any doubt about the plane being dissected, further dissection in the base of the incision may be needed. The incision is extended until the surgeon feels comfortable that the fibroid can be removed. Generally, fibroids will begin to extrude somewhat when the incision is of the appropriate length. Bleeding, not generally a problem during this step, is controlled with bipolar

[150]

cautery. The fibroid is then grasped through either of the lower quadrant trocar sheaths using a toothed forceps. Forceps have been found preferable to the use of a myoma screw since the fibroid can be quickly grasped and regrasped, changing the position of the fibroid relative to the other dissecting instruments to allow more rapid dissection. The contralateral lower quadrant sheath is used to carry an atraumatic grasping forceps to hold the myometrium or serosa of the uterus, and, using traction and countertraction, the fibroid is dissected from the myometrial bed using hook scissors through the midline trocar sheath. The scissors may be used bluntly or sharply depending on the presence of fibrous bands. Vascular bands that are encountered are treated with bipolar cautery prior to division. The toothed grasping forceps is then moved to the opposite lower quadrant trocar sheath and the opposite side of the myoma is dissected free. As the base of the myoma comes into view, any vessels present are treated with bipolar cautery prior to division. The myoma is then completely separated from the uterus and left in the peritoneal cavity while the uterine defect is closed.

If the myoma was subserosal or extremely superficial intramural in location, the serosa and any involved myometrium may be closed in one layer using 4-0 polydioxanone (PDS; Ethicon, Somerville, NJ) on a small straight needle (Ethicon Z-420) and tying extracorporeally with a laparoscopic knot pusher (Clarke-Reich Ligator; Marlow Surgical Technologies, Willoughby, OH) (Figure 12-1). Deeper intramural fibroids require layered closure of the myometrium. The technique described by Reich is used (13). A suture of 0 polyglactin 910 on a CT 1 or CT 2 needle is introduced into the abdominal cavity as shown in Figures 12-2 to 12-5. Two layers are usually sufficient to close the myometrium. Interrupted simple sutures are placed, ligated with half-hitches using the laparoscopic knot pusher. Following closure of the myometrium, the serosa is closed as noted previously. If possible, the serosal sutures should be placed in inverted fashion to allow the knot to remain below the peritoneum.

The myoma is now removed either by colpotomy, removal through a suprapubic minilaparotomy incision, or fragmentation using a commer-

CHAPTER 12
Laparoscopic Myomectomy

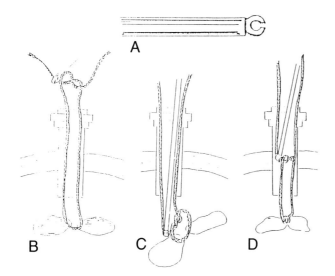

Figure 12-1 (A) Clarke knot-pusher. (B) Application to a single tie. (C) The first throw of the knot is passed through the trapless trocar sleeve. (D) The second throw is passed through the trocar sleeve to secure the first. Reprinted with permission from the American College of Obstetricians and Gynecologists (Obstet Gynecol 1992;79(1):143–147.)

[151]

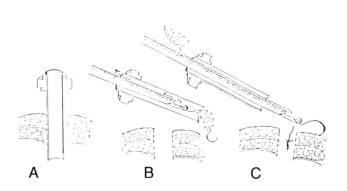

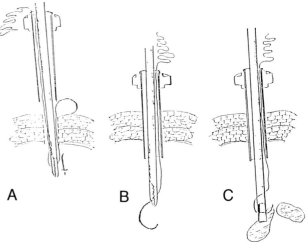

Figure 12-2 (A) Short trocar sleeve in place. (B) Distal suture is loaded into the sleeve removed from the peritoneal cavity. (C) The suture is grasped 3 cm from the curved needle. Reprinted with permission from the American College of Obstetricians and Gynecologists (Obstet Gynecol 1992;79(1):143–147.)

Figure 12-3 (A) Needle-holder is directed back through the original incision. (B) The sleeve is replaced over the needle-holder. (C) Suture is applied with the curved needle-holder. Reprinted with permission from the American College of Obstetricians and Gynecologists (Obstet Gynecol 1992;79:143–147.)

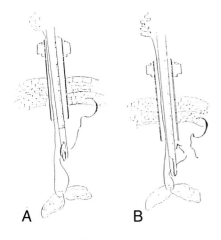

Figure 12-4 (A) Suture is cut 3 cm from the needle. (B) The cut end is pulled through the trocar sleeve and the needle is placed in the parietal peritoneum. Reprinted with permission from the American College of Obstetricians and Gynecologists (Obstet Gynecol 1992;79(1):143–147.)

Figure 12-5 (A) Knot placement. (B) The needle end is retrieved. (C) The needle is removed from the peritoneal cavity after withdrawing the trocar sleeve, which is then replaced. Reprinted with permission from the American College of Obstetricians and Gynecologists (Obstet Gynecol 1992;79(1):143–147.)

cially available SEMM tissue morcellator (WISAP, West Germany). Large fibroids over 4 cm are divided into segments prior to removal through a colpotomy or suprapubic incision. A colpotomy can be made by placing a sponge stick in the posterior vaginal fornix and visualizing the bulge laparoscopically anterior to the sigmoid and medial to both uterosacral ligaments. The cul-de-sac is then opened with laparoscopic scissors or unipolar cautery. The tissue is removed and the colpotomy closed vaginally with a continuous absorbable suture.

If a minilaparotomy is performed, a 2½- to 3-cm incision is made through the skin and fascia. The segments of fibroid are directed to the incision and pulled out with a 10-mm grasper or Kocher forceps. The minilaparotomy fascial incision is closed with continuous absorbable suture and the pelvis irrigated and inspected for hemostasis. If there are small bleeding points noted on the uterine serosa, these may be controlled with figure-eight sutures of 4-0 polydioxanone. Reinfiltration

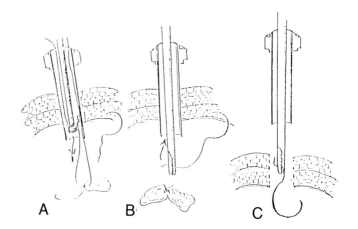

with the vasopressin solution is rarely necessary. If hemostasis is questionable, a 5-mm flexible drain may be left in the pelvis, placed through the lateral lower quadrant trocar and directed into the cul-de-sac with grasping forceps. The trocar sheath is then removed from the incision, leaving the drain in place. Output from this drain can be monitored for 6–8 hours, and, if low, the drain may then be removed.

Patients are discharged within 23 hours of admission and may return to full activity within three to seven days. In the case of a colpotomy, the patient should refrain from intercourse for approximately six weeks.

Complications

No prospective study has, as yet, addressed the issue of complications of laparoscopic myomectomy relative to those encountered at the time of myomectomy by the abdominal route. Specifically, the risk of adhesion formation after laparoscopic myomectomy needs to be addressed as well as concerns about the structural integrity of the uterus following laparoscopic closure of the myometrium.

Discussion

For selected patients with symptomatic uterine fibroids, laparoscopic myomectomy is a reasonable alternative to laparotomy. The surgeon's level of expertise with endoscopic surgical procedures is of paramount importance in determining which patients are candidates for laparoscopic myomectomy. Desire for future childbearing should remain a relative contraindication to laparoscopic myomectomy until further information concerning adhesion formation and subsequent pregnancy outcome is collected.

References

1 Mattingly RF, Thompson JD. TeLinde's operative gynecology. Philadelphia: JB Lippincott Co, 1985;647–663.
2 Buttram VC, Reiter RC. Uterine leiomyomata: etiology, symptomatology, and management. Fertil Steril 1981;36:433–445.
3 Verkauf BS. Myomectomy for fertility enhancement and preservation. Fertil Steril 1992;58:1–15.
4 Smith DC, Uhlir JK. Myomectomy as a reproductive procedure. Am J Obstet Gynecol 1990;162:1476–1482.
5 Daniell JF, Gurley LD. Laparoscopic treatment of clinically significant symptomatic uterine fibroids. J Gynecol Surg 1991;7:37–40.
6 Dubuisson JB, Lecura F, Foulot H, Mandelbrot L, Aubriot FX, Mouly M. Myomectomy by laparoscopy: a preliminary report of 43 cases. Fertil Steril 1991;56:827–830.
7 Nezhat C, Nezhat F, Silfen SL, Schaffer N, Evans D. Laparoscopic myomectomy. Int J Fertil 1991;36:275–280.
8 The American Fertility Society. Guideline for practice: myomas and reproductive dysfunction. The American Fertility Society, Birmingham, Alabama 1992.
9 Harris WJ. Uterine dehiscence following laparoscopic myomectomy. Obstet Gynecol 1992;80[3 (Pt 2)]:545–546.
10 Leibsohn S, d'Ablaing G, Mishell DR, Schlaerth JB. Leiomyosarcoma in a series of hysterectomies performed for presumed uterine leiomyomas. Am J Obstet Gynecol 1990;162:968–976.

[153]

11 Friedman AJ, Rein MS, Harrison-Atlas D, Garfield JM, Doubilet PM. A randomized, placebo-controlled, double-blind study evaluating leuprolide acetate depot treatment before myomectomy. Fertil Steril 1989;52:728–733.

12 Friedman AJ, Fine C, Rein MS, Daly M, Juneau-Norcross M. Recurrence of myomas after myomectomy in women pretreated with leuprolide acetate depot or placebo. Fertil Steril 1992;58:205–208.

13 Reich H, Clarke HC, Sekel L. A simple method for ligating with straight and curved needles in operative laparoscopy. Obstet Gynecol 1992;79:143–147.

13 Hysteroscopic Myomectomy

ALAN S. PENZIAS & ALAN H. DECHERNEY

Whereas nearly all areas of gynecologic surgery have been adapted or modified through the application of endoscopy, the endoscopic treatment of uterine leiomyomata leads in the development of previously undescribed procedures. A good example of an endoscopic procedure recapitulating a classic open abdominal technique is the treatment of ectopic pregnancy. If a salpingectomy is performed at laparotomy, the surgeon clamps, cuts, and ties the vascular attachment of the affected fallopian tube and excises the specimen. While the endoscopic instrumentation used to perform a salpingectomy differs somewhat to accommodate the laparoscopic approach, the technique is remarkably similar. Grasping instruments hold the fallopian tube in place while the vessels and ligamentous supports are severed. Hemostasis is achieved with cautery, surgical clips, or suture ligatures. In contrast, hysteroscopic myomectomy bears only a limited resemblance to the time-honored abdominal approach. The attendant morbidity of abdominal myomectomy for fibroids that are amenable to hysteroscopic treatment vis-à-vis duration of hospitalization, term of postoperative disability, potential for adhesion formation, and the need for cesarean section should pregnancy ensue has been virtually eliminated.

While the earliest series describing the hysteroscopic resection of submucous uterine fibroids dates back to 1976 (1), the vast majority of the literature on this topic has appeared only in the past five years. When appraising the data and experience regarding hysteroscopic myomectomy, one must bear in mind its relative youth compared to the traditional abdominal approach. In fact, the magnitude of the difference is best appreciated when one considers that the first abdominal myomectomy was attributed to W.L. Atlee in 1844 (2). The difference in experience, which approaches 150 years, implies that the evolution of the hysteroscopic approach to the treatment of submucous uterine fibroids is still in its nascence. The indications for surgery, operative techniques, therapeutic endpoints, and treatment outcomes continue to change as the collective experience grows and as different forms of instrumentation are developed to meet the changing needs.

This chapter will review the current indications, preoperative evaluation, surgical techniques, and outcomes of hysteroscopic myomectomy. We will also attempt to clearly label our own surgical preferences when discussing methods and do not imply that these practices are the only acceptable techniques.

Indications for hysteroscopic myomectomy

The most common patient complaints that lead to a thorough evaluation and culminate with hysteroscopic myomectomy are abnormal vaginal bleeding and reproductive failure. Dysfunctional uterine bleeding is a nonspecific hallmark of a structural or hormonal abnormality. The evaluation of the problem is best done in the context of the specific historical and physical characteristics of the patient seeking treatment. When the etiology of the aberrant bleeding is unclear even after a comprehensive hormonal evaluation and physical examination and/or medical therapy has failed to correct the problem, additional diagnostic studies of the uterus are indicated. It has been our experience that some women with a normal-sized uterus by bimanual examination will harbor one or more submucous uterine fibroids. When these fibroids are resected, normal menstrual function is restored.

Reproductive failure in the context of uterine fibroids encompasses patients with primary or secondary infertility as well as recurrent pregnancy loss. During the comprehensive evaluation of such patients, anatomic evaluation of the uterus is warranted. If the evaluation of the uterine anatomy reveals the presence of uterine fibroids, the treating physician must consider their location and determine the likelihood that they are contributing to the reproductive dilemma. The contribution of intramural and subserosal myomas to reproductive failure in some circumstances is tenuous at best. Furthermore, the abdominal approach to myomectomy may engender complications that further perturb the reproductive process. In contrast, a good case can be made for the direct causality between virtually all submucous fibroids and reproductive failure. The apparent relationship between submucous fibroids and poor reproductive outcome should be tempered with the understanding that discovery of such pathology should not truncate the comprehensive evaluation of infertility or recurrent pregnancy loss, as other significant contributing factors may coexist. Failure to discover possible concomitant factors may result in delayed, incomplete, or inappropriate therapy.

Contraindications to hysteroscopic myomectomy

It is worth mentioning at this point that there may be instances where asymptomatic submucous fibroids are discovered incidentally during the investigation of an entirely unrelated problem. Typically, the leiomyomata are revealed by a pelvic ultrasound or MRI scan while a patient is being evaluated for a urologic, gastrointestinal, or neurologic malady. There is no literature to date that supports prophylactic surgical intervention in these cases. A less distinct issue is that of pelvic pain. While it is true that pelvic pain has been attributed to degenerating leiomyomas, this condition rarely occurs spontaneously. Degeneration of uterine fibroids occurs most commonly in pregnancy, though it has been reported

[156]

following gonadotropin-releasing hormone (GnRH) agonist administration (3,4) and with the use of oral contraceptives (5). Coexisting pelvic pathology, including adenomyosis, endometriosis, and pelvic inflammatory disease, further clouds the relationship between pelvic pain and uterine fibroids. At the present time, it appears that hysteroscopic myomectomy alone does not have a significant role in the treatment of patients with pelvic pain.

The role of hysteroscopy in the treatment of prolapsed pedunculated submucous fibroids warrants discussion. Traditionally, these fibroids have been treated with simple vaginal myomectomy (6). Frequently performed without anesthesia, the stalk is ligated and allowed to retract into the uterine cavity. One study reported on a series of 46 women with symptomatic prolapsed pedunculated submucous myomas. Vaginal myomectomy was successful in 43 and failed in three patients, necessitating abdominal operation. Only 8.8% of 34 patients with a median follow-up of 5.5 years required repeat vaginal myomectomy, and only 5.9% needed hysterectomy (7). The major difficulty in applying hysteroscopy to this condition is that the cervical dilation that permits passage of the myoma into the vagina hampers one's ability to instill and maintain a distending medium in the uterine cavity (Figure 13-1). Furthermore, replacement of the myoma risks bringing a large number of bacteria into the uterine cavity without any clear therapeutic advantage. When uterine preservation is the chief goal, removal of the bulk of the myoma may be performed vaginally, with consideration given to an interval hysteroscopy after the cervix has had time to reconstitute to its original state. If this is not technically feasible, an abdominal approach should be contemplated.

Finally, some authors quote size limits for uterine fibroids above which endoscopic surgery should not be attempted. With regard to hysteroscopy in specific, there are no convincing data upon which to base such a recommendation. The chief limiting factors appear to be related to the surgical experience of the operator, the anatomic configuration of the myoma in question, and the quantity and type of distention media being utilized.

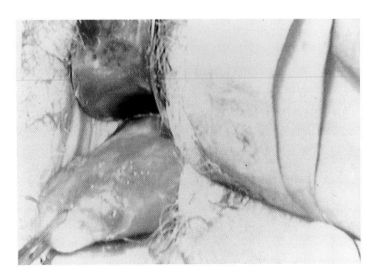

Figure 13-1 Vaginal myomectomy for a prolapsed pedunculated submucous fibroid.

Preoperative imaging studies

The diagnosis of submucous uterine fibroids is often not made definitively until the time of an operative procedure. Preoperative diagnosis may be aided by several imaging modalities, including hysterosalpingography (HSG), ultrasonography (US) and magnetic resonance imaging (MRI). Preoperative imaging studies can aid in planning appropriate therapy by determining the size, number, and, frequently, the location of uterine fibroids. The choice of which modality to employ is often determined by the availability of specific resources, taking into account the relative expense of each test. In an attempt to define the sensitivity, specificity, and accuracy of the various imaging modalities, one group of investigators compared preoperative localization of uterine fibroids with MRI versus US and HSG (8). Eleven women with a history of infertility and uterine leiomyomas underwent MRI of the pelvis prior to myomectomy. Nine patients also had a preoperative pelvic US and ten also had a preoperative HSG. Among the nine patients who underwent both MRI and US, the sensitivity (85%) and accuracy (94%) of MRI was significantly better than that of US (sensitivity = 69%; accuracy = 87%). For the ten patients who underwent both MRI and HSG, the sensitivity (91%) and accuracy (96%) of MRI was better than that of HSG (sensitivity = 18%; accuracy = 72%). No direct comparison was made between US and HSG. The specificities of the three modalities did not significantly differ (100%, 97%, and 98% for MRI, US, and HSG, respectively), that is, fibroids identified by preoperative imaging were nearly always confirmed histologically to be fibroids. This small study appears to confirm an otherwise intuitive impression that the sensitivity of MRI (~88%) for diagnosing and localizing uterine fibroids is higher than that of either US (69%) or HSG (18%). These results call into question the utility of HSG in identifying and localizing uterine fibroids. Another group of investigators studied 34 patients entering a program of in vitro fertilization. Each patient had evidence of a normal endometrial cavity by HSG, but 43% had a visible abnormality at the time of hysteroscopy (9). Others have reported discordance between the HSG and hysteroscopy at a rate approaching 30% (10). In our institution, the least expensive of the three modalities is an US, followed closely by an HSG. Each of these is significantly less costly than an MRI scan. Taken together, we conclude that US is the screening procedure of choice for identifying and localizing uterine fibroids because of its high sensitivity, widespread availability, safety, and relatively low cost. When other uterine pathology is suspected or the US is indeterminate, MRI should be considered the next imaging step (11).

Preoperative evaluation and counseling

As in any procedure, proper patient selection is the first step in reducing complications. For example, patients with extremely large fibroids, as estimated by preoperative imaging, may benefit from intraoperative conversion to an abdominal myomectomy or even hysterectomy. Anticipation of this possibility allows the patient to give true informed consent to the expected procedures and affords the surgeon maximum intra-operative flexibility. A risk-benefit assessment must be made for each specific patient. Choosing the appropriate setting for the performance of the procedure is important. A patient with significant coexisting medical conditions or in whom there is some likelihood of intraoperative conversion to laparotomy might be better served by having a hysteroscopy in a hospital setting. However, many patients who are appropriately selected may do extremely well in outpatient surgical care centers.

Potential adverse outcomes, both major and minor, are best discussed with the patient well in advance of the procedure. In operative hysteroscopy, these include bleeding, uterine perforation, fluid overload, infection, and embolism. These issues will be addressed later in this chapter.

Surgery

Instrumentation

The variety of hysteroscopes currently on the market are tailored to many different applications. Flexible instruments and traditional ones of narrow outer diameter are primarily intended for purely diagnostic purposes. With hysteroscopes of larger widths (8–10 mm outer diameter), visualization of the endometrial cavity can be accomplished by direct inspection, or a magnified image can be projected in crisp, clear detail. These instruments have the advantage of maintaining optical integrity while introducing operative instruments. In addition, some instrument designs enable continuous laminar flow of distention media in order to sustain the clarity of the operative field. Maintenance of a transparent operative field is especially important in cases where bleeding is likely to occur.

Operative instruments have been designed for hysteroscopic use to facilitate a range of desired procedures. When the goal is ablation of the endometrium, a roller-bar or ball can be employed; this procedure is described in greater detail in Chapter 14. The loop electrode, or re-sectoscope, is a versatile tool that can be used in numerous procedures. The resectoscope is particularly useful in resection of submucous uterine fibroids. Knife electrodes concentrate cutting or coagulating current into a high-energy tip. Because the surface area of the knife electrode is small, the power density at the tip is higher for a given voltage setting than, for example, is the roller ball or roller bar.

Fiberoptic lasers afford another approach to hysteroscopic surgery. The Nd:YAG (neodymium-yttrium-aluminum-garnet), KTP (potassium-titanyl-phosphate), and argon lasers are all well suited for hysteroscopic use. Unlike the CO_2 laser, which cannot pass through fluids, the Nd:YAG, argon, and KTP lasers are able to pass through flexible fibers and fluids. The wavelengths of the argon and KTP lasers, 0.458–0.515 μM and 0.532 μM, respectively, make them most amenable to absorption by darkly pigmented tissue. These lasers will penetrate tissue 1–2 mm

[159]

with minimal scatter and can be used for their cutting action. The Nd:YAG laser wavelength of 1.064 μM allows it to pass deeply into tissue before it is absorbed (12). The Nd:YAG wave will scatter upon contact with tissue, making it a poor cutting instrument but an excellent coagulator. However, the use of a sculpted sapphire tip can focus the beam and allow it to function as a laser scalpel.

Traditional instruments, such as scissors, biopsy forceps, and graspers have also been adapted for hysteroscopic use.

Intrauterine visualization

The success of operative hysteroscopy is dependent upon the ability to deliver light to the uterine cavity and visualize its surface. Fiberoptic technology enables high intensity light to travel from its point of origin through a flexible cable into the hysteroscope. The light must then pass out of the hysteroscope into the medium used to distend the uterine cavity. The optical principle that forms the foundation of fiberoptics rests upon the index of refraction of the fiber carrying the light wave. Light-carrying fibers are constructed of a variety of materials designed to adjust the fiber's index of refraction. Materials whose index of refraction is higher than the surrounding environment will reflect light waves within its confines internally, and none of the light will be reflected outward. A focusing lens is placed at the end of the light cable, which allows the light to escape from the fibers and directs it into the hysteroscope. The optics of the hysteroscope are designed to vary the focal length of the instrument such that the illuminated uterine cavity can be adequately visualized. The index of refraction of the selected distention medium will also affect the visual field. CO_2 has an index of refraction (IR) of 1.00, whereas the IR of saline solution is 1.37 and that of high molecular weight dextran is 1.39. These indices mean that CO_2 will afford a wider field of view and lower magnification than will a liquid medium (13). CO_2 is not used during hysteroscopic myomectomy because of the risk of introducing a CO_2 bubble under high pressure into an open blood vessel, resulting in pulmonary embolism.

Fluid media in common use include saline, Ringer's lactate, glycine, sorbitol, and high molecular weight dextran. Electrolyte-containing solutions are not compatible with operative hysteroscopy where electrosurgical instruments will be used. This is because these liquids act as conductors of the electrical current. In addition, low viscosity fluids are miscible with blood. The operative field afforded by these liquids is obscured rapidly with the addition of even small amounts of flowing blood. These limits, along with their ready availability and low cost, make them more suitable for diagnostic procedures. Dextran has the advantage of being immiscible with blood, and it does not conduct electricity. These characteristics are compatible with operative procedures, especially where bleeding may be anticipated.

[160]

Pedunculated intrauterine fibroids

When a pedunculated uterine fibroid is encountered at the time of hysteroscopy, its point of attachment to the uterine wall should be examined (Figure 13-2). The pertinent features that should be noted include its point of insertion, the thickness of the stalk, and degree of vascularity visible on the surface of the stalk. The point of attachment is an important consideration because those with low lateral insertion may lie close to high-pressure uterine vessels. Vigorous dissection or inadvertent avulsion may lead to serious hemorrhage. The stalk diameter and degree of superficial vascularization will help guide the operative approach.

If the stalk connecting the myoma and the uterine wall is thin and tenuous in appearance, hysteroscopic scissors with or without cautery may be used. Selective cautery then may be applied as needed. The now free-floating myoma can be removed either by undirected passage of forceps into the uterine cavity or by morcellation and removal in pieces. Where the stalk is thick or vascular, hemostasis is best maintained by an instrument that coagulates as it bisects the tissue. Examples include scissors attached to an electrocautery device and the resectoscope loop. The knife electrode or fiberoptic laser with sculpted scalpel tip are optimal for these conditions. These instruments concentrate cutting or coagulating current into a high-energy tip. Because the surface area of these tools is small, the power density at the tip is higher for a given voltage setting than is the resectoscope loop or unfocused laser beam.

Sessile submucous uterine fibroids

The degree of protrusion of the myoma into the uterine cavity will often portend the volume of myoma that remains intramural. Enucleation of

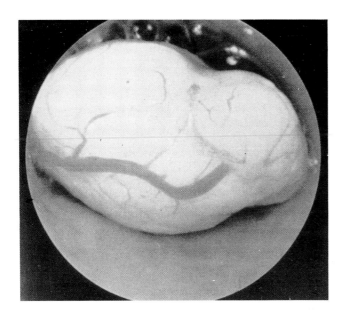

Figure 13-2 Large pedunculated submucous myoma.

the entire myoma can be achieved if the mass is predominantly submucous. Several techniques have been described, including the use of the resectoscope loop, enucleation with scissors (1,14), induction of necrosis or vaporization with Nd:YAG laser (15), and transection into pieces with a fiberoptic laser terminating in a sapphire tip (16). Scissors are most suited to removal of small myomas as it is difficult to morcellate a larger fibroid with them. Laser vaporization is impractical and time-consuming for anything other than extremely small fibroids. Passage of a sapphire-tipped laser scalpel through the myoma may be difficult as the device may deviate from the desired plane of transection as it is advanced through the fibroid. Scissors and the laser scalpel are also easiest to use if the fibroid protrudes at an angle perpendicular to the plane of the instrument. Fundal myoma insertions are more challenging to resect with these instruments, and the risk of inadvertent perforation is increased.

We prefer the use of the resectoscope loop. Using this instrument, the myoma is shaved into fragments that can be easily removed. The technique that we employ begins by extending the resectoscope loop beyond the myoma and slowly retracting it until contact with the myoma is made. Once firm contact is made, electrical current is applied and the loop is slowly retracted toward the hysteroscope (Figure 13-3). Slow retraction is essential, as it permits the loop to heat to maximum cutting temperature so that it can bore through the myoma while passing in the direction of the hysteroscope. Rapid retraction will cut only a shallow path, thereby increasing the number of passes necessary to resect the myoma and creating a larger number of myoma fragments. An increase in the number of passes required to resect the fibroid increases operative time, and the larger number of fragments obscures the surgical field.

By placing the loop behind the fibroid and gently retracting toward the hysteroscope before current is applied, we are able to visualize the relationship of the fibroid to the uterine walls and make any necessary adjustments in position before cutting. The retraction of the hot resectoscope loop toward the hysteroscope ensures that there is a clear and visible path at all times. This action virtually eliminates the risk of uterine perforation during that portion of the operation.

Figure 13-3 Resectoscope loop resection of a sessile submucous uterine fibroid.

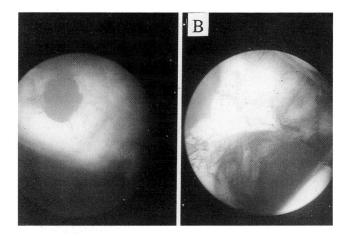

When a large portion of the myoma is intramural, a practical surgical compromise is to resect the accessible portion of the myoma until it is flush with the remaining surfaces of the uterine cavity. It is not feasible with current techniques to safely resect that portion of a myoma that is primarily intramural. The risks of attempting complete removal of an intramural myoma include uterine perforation, hemorrhage, and creation of a weak point in the uterine wall. The degree of risk is likely to be proportional to the size and position of the remaining myoma; however, specific parameters have not been adequately quantified in the literature to date.

If, during the procedure, the field becomes irreversibly obscured, whether due to a large number of myoma fragments or blood, it is better to terminate the procedure and return at a later date, if necessary, than continue blindly. If a significant portion of the offending myoma has been resected prior to cessation of the procedure, necrosis at the cauterized base, which remains in situ, will often effect its spontaneous recession, obviating the need for further surgery. Alternatively, the much reduced base may be covered by normal endometrium. If the presenting complaint returns, then a second hysteroscopic procedure can be performed.

The role of GnRH agonist

GnRH agonists are known to diminish total uterine volume and intraoperative blood loss in large myomatous uteri subjected to abdominal myomectomy (17). In addition, their use will arrest bleeding and allow the anemic patient to build a reserve prior to surgery. However, it has been reported that use of the agonist in small uteri may not reduce blood loss significantly and may obscure the presence of smaller fibroids, which escape removal and result in short-term recurrence, thereby limiting the efficacy of the surgery (18). There are several case reports where GnRH agonist therapy palliated the presenting symptoms and delayed definitive surgical therapy of a leiomyosarcoma (19). However, the incidence of leiomyosarcoma in uterine leiomyomas is extremely rare and is estimated to be between 0.13 to 0.29% (20).

The evidence for GnRH agonist administration in hysteroscopic myomectomy is scant. One prospective study reported a reduction in the operating time, bleeding during the operation, and the amount of distention medium required after depot leuprolide acetate administration (21). The benefit from a period of amenorrhea in the anemic patient awaiting hysteroscopic myomectomy is certain. However, it remains to be seen whether the long-term postoperative outcomes, especially in patients with reproductive failure, are equivalent for patients with and without preoperative GnRH agonist therapy.

Complications

Bleeding

Immediately after removal of the hysteroscope, the uterus will contract to expel the distending medium, blood, and any particulate matter. If bleeding following expulsion of this material persists, it can often be treated by the placement in the uterine cavity of a 30 ml Foley catheter balloon filled with 15 to 30 ml of saline. Normal uterine contraction around the balloon will often tamponade bleeding surfaces. Once tamponaded, platelet plug formation will occur, followed by activation of the coagulation cascade. Some patients may find an over-distended balloon quite uncomfortable, so its volume should be titrated between hemostasis and patient tolerance. In our experience, the balloon can remain in place up to 72 hours before it is removed. In such cases, we elect to place the patient on prophylactic antibiotics for the duration of catheter placement. The length of time that the balloon remains in place is dependent upon rate of bleeding and other clinical considerations. Patient acceptance of an intrauterine balloon is significantly enhanced if they are counseled about the possibility preoperatively. Placement of the balloon does not mean that the patient must be admitted for in-hospital observation. However, daily interaction, in person or by telephone, between patient and physician is optimal until the balloon is removed.

In rare circumstances, postoperative hemorrhage reflects a systemic coagulopathy brought about most commonly when high molecular weight dextran is used for uterine distention. The clinical recognition of this rare etiology is bleeding at sites distant from the uterus.

Uterine perforation

Physical examination and determination of uterine flexion prior to placement of the hysteroscope is essential. Passage of a uterine sound with assessment of the uterine cavity depth can further aid in the procedure. Significant anteflexion or retroflexion increases the risk of perforation. Forcing the hysteroscope through an inadequately dilated cervix further increases the risk. While perforation in the midline generally does not have significant sequelae and does not routinely mandate laparoscopic inspection, lateral perforation poses the risk of lacerating major uterine vessels. Laparoscopy and direct visualization of the perforation site may be quite useful in the case of a lateral perforation. If perforation occurs, it is advisable to discontinue the operative procedure and return at a later date. If the uterus is perforated with an operative instrument, particularly an electrosurgical or laser instrument, there is a risk of injury to the bowel or bladder. When the surgeon's index of suspicion for bowel injury is low, observation may suffice with the understanding that thermal injury to the bowel with subsequent leakage of intestinal contents will not be manifest for seven to ten days. When injury to the bowel or mesentery is suspected, inspection of the site is indicated. Some physicians, with advanced endoscopic training and skills, may be able to adequately visualize these structures laparoscopically. In lieu of such experience, an exploratory laparotomy may be necessary. If a bowel injury has occurred, appropriate surgical consultation should be obtained and a repair initiated.

Fluid overload

Absorption of glycine, sorbitol, or high molecular weight dextran, especially during lengthy operative procedures, can result in significant fluid overload. The entry of dextran into the circulation can produce pulmonary edema or hyponatremia. While no more than 500 ml of this material should be used during operative hysteroscopy, smaller volumes can still induce complications (22). Monitoring input and overflow volumes of distention media is useful in assessing patient absorption. If the operative procedure requires long periods of time and large volumes of distention media, intraoperative monitoring of serum electrolytes is advisable.

Infection

Infection following hysteroscopic myomectomy is rare. Preoperative determination of upper or lower genital infection can frequently avoid significant complications. Despite the fact that dextran is a compound of polymerized sucrose, infection following the use of this distention medium in a previously uninfected patient is uncommon.

Embolism

The risk of embolism is dramatically reduced by not using CO_2 during hysteroscopic myomectomy. Dextran embolism can occur and may be manifested by disseminated intravascular coagulopathy. Fortunately, this complication is a rare occurrence.

Outcome

In contrast to myomectomy at laparotomy, hysteroscopic myomectomy decreases the direct and indirect morbidity associated with the procedure. It is most commonly performed on an outpatient basis and, therefore, does not routinely require a hospital stay. The common endpoints of success are elimination of dysmenorrhea, absence of menorrhagia, and pregnancy. One study of 92 consecutive patients having resectoscopic myomectomy over a three-year period reported elimination of dysmenorrhea in 86% and absence of menorrhagia in 81% of the patients. Of the 13 patients desiring pregnancy, ten (77%) succeeded, with two miscarriages in a total of 11 gestations (23). In general, the first clinical results of hysteroscopic treatment seem satisfactory, with average success rates of 85%. However, information about the long-term outcome for the majority of the reported cases is not available (24). An encouraging sign of long-term outcome is foreshadowed by the one study with lengthy follow-up that demonstrated an 84% cure rate in 94 patients who were followed for nine years after hysteroscopic myomectomy (25).

While large numbers of patients have undergone hysteroscopic myomectomy, no randomized trials have been conducted (26). Despite this limitation, hysteroscopy offers perhaps the least invasive approach to symptomatic submucous uterine fibroids.

References

1 Neuwirth RS, Amin HK. Excision of submucous fibroids with hysteroscopic control. Am J Obstet Gynecol 1976;126:95–99.

2 Verkauf BS. Myomectomy for fertility enhancement and preservation. Fertil Steril 1992;58:1–15.

3 Chipato T, Healy DL, Vollenhoven B, Buckler HM. Pelvic pain complicating LHRH analogue treatment of fibroids. Aust N Z J Obstet Gynaecol 1991;31:383–384.

4 Chang MY, Tsai FB, Soong YK. Infarcted intramural uterine leiomyomata during buserelin acetate treatment. Chang Keng I Hsueh 1993;16:129–132.

5 Myles JL, Hart WR. Apoplectic leiomyomas of the uterus. A clinicopathologic study of five distinctive hemorrhagic leiomyomas associated with oral contraceptive usage. Am J Surg Pathol 1985;9:798–805.

6 Brooks GG, Stage AH. The surgical management of prolapsed pedunculated submucous leiomyomas. Surg Gynecol Obstet 1975;141:397–398.

7 Ben-Baruch G, Schiff E, Menashe Y, Menczer J. Immediate and late outcome of vaginal myomectomy for prolapsed pedunculated submucous myoma. Obstet Gynecol 1988;72:858–861.

8 Dudiak CM, Turner DA, Patel SK, Archie JT, Silver B, Norusis M. Uterine leiomyomas in the infertile patient: preoperative localization with MR imaging versus US and hysterosalpingography. Radiology 1988;167:627–630.

9 Shamma FN, Lee G, Gutmann JN, Lavy G. The role of office hysteroscopy in in vitro fertilization. Fertil Steril 1992;58:1237–1239.

10 Taylor PJ, Goswamy RK. Hysteroscopy in infertility and habitual abortion. Hum Reprod 1989;4:13–16.

11 Scoutt LM, McCarthy SM. Applications of magnetic resonance imaging to gynecology. Top Magn Reson Imaging 1990;2:37–49.

12 Laser Technology. ACOG Technical Bulletin 146. American College of Obstetricians and Gynecologists, Washington, DC, September, 1990.

13 Seigler AM, Kemmann E. Hysteroscopy. Obstet Gynecol Survey 1975;30:567–588.

14 Valle RF. Hysteroscopic removal of submucous leiomyomas. J Gynecol Surg 1990;6:89–96.

15 Baggish MS, Sze EHM, Morgan G. Hysteroscopic treatment of symptomatic submucous myomata uteri with the Nd:Yag laser. J Gynecol Surg 1989;5:27–36.

16 Loffer FD. Removal of large symptomatic intrauterine growths by the hysteroscopic resectoscope. Obstet Gynecology 1990;76:836–840.

17 Friedman AJ, Rein MS, Harrison-Atlas D, Garfield JM, Doubilet PM. A randomized, placebo-controlled, double-blind study evaluating leuprolide acetate depot treatment before myomectomy. Fertil Steril 1989;52:728–733.

18 Fedele L, Vercellini P, Bianchi S, Brioschi D, Dorta M. Treatment with GnRH agonists before myomectomy and the risk of short-term myoma recurrence. Br J Obstet Gynaecol 1990;97:393–396.

19 Murphy NJ, Wallace DL. Gonadotropin-releasing hormone (GnRH) agonist therapy for reduction of leiomyoma volume. Gynecol Oncol 1993;49:266–267.

20 Leibsohn S, d'Ablaing G, Mishell DR Jr, Schlaerth JB. Leiomyosarcoma in a series of hysterectomies performed for presumed uterine leiomyomas. Am J Obstet Gynecol 1990;162:968–974.

21 Perino A, Chianchiano N, Petronio M, Cittadini E. Role of leuprolide acetate depot in hysteroscopic surgery: a controlled study. Fertil Steril 1993;59:507–510.

22 McLucas B. Hyskon complications in hysteroscopic surgery. Obstet Gynecol Survey 1991;46:196–200.

23 Corson SL, Brooks PG. Resectoscopic myomectomy. Fertil Steril 1991;55:1041–1044.

24 Grainger DA, DeCherney AH. Hysteroscopic management of uterine bleeding. Baillieres Clin Obstet Gynaecol 1989;3:403–414.

25 Derman SG, Rehnstrom J, Neuwirth RS. The long-term effectiveness of hysteroscopic treatment of menorrhagia and leiomyomas. Obstet Gynecol 1991;77:591–594.

26 de Wit A. Hysteroscopy: an evolving case of minimally invasive therapy in gynaecology. Health Policy 1993;23:113–124.

14 Endometrial Ablation as an Alternative to Hysterectomy

JAMES F. DANIELL

Excessive menstrual blood loss in the latter part of a woman's reproductive years accounts for an important portion of the large number of hysterectomies being performed today. Once malignancy or other organic lesions have been ruled out, dysfunctional uterine bleeding is diagnosed. Despite the theoretical ability to control the bleeding with one of many medical regimens, patient dissatisfaction with these agents often ultimately leads to hysterectomy. Although mortality from hysterectomy for benign disorders is low, short-term morbidity may be as high as 43% (1). There is also considerable concern with respect to the long-term sequelae of hysterectomy, which may include premature loss of ovarian function, psychosexual problems, and urinary tract symptoms (2). In addition, the costs of the procedure and hospital stay are high. Prolonged postoperative recovery periods remove many women from the work force and, thus, create additional costs to society.

Ever since Asherman (3,4) described post-traumatic uterine adhesion formation resulting in hypomenorrhea or amenorrhea, gynecologists have looked for methods to destroy the endometrial lining to control excessive menstrual blood loss. The use of radiofrequency-induced thermal ablation using a nonvisual transcervical method may prove to be successful in the future as a minimally invasive approach to ablation of the endometrium (5).

Recent advances in hysteroscopic technique now appear to offer an effective, less invasive, and certainly less costly approach to the management of dysfunctional uterine bleeding than hysterectomy (6). This chapter reviews current information on endometrial destruction by Nd:YAG laser and the resectoscope as definitive therapy for menorrhagia to allow patients to avoid hysterectomy.

History

Endometrial ablation has evolved by bringing together two observations: the recognition that destruction of the endometrium will cause amenorrhea and the ability to visualize and operate within the uterine cavity. In 1894, Fritsch (7) recognized the correlation between post-traumatic uterine adhesion formation and amenorrhea. The syndrome was more carefully described following World War II and named in honor of Asherman (3,4).

Early attempts to induce this condition deliberately to control bleeding included the instillation of such agents as quinacrine, methyl-cyanoacrylate, oxacilic acid, and paraformaldehyde. The introduction of superheated steam, a technique of cryocoagulation, and the use of intracavity radium all were briefly in vogue (8). The unreliability of results and potential risks led to the abandonment of all of these procedures. These approaches failed because of the tremendous capacity of the endometrium to regenerate. It is now apparent that unless the basal layer of the endometrium is destroyed, regeneration will be inevitable in most cases.

The first visualization of the uterine cavity was performed by Pantaleoni in 1869. He used a cystoscope, which recently had been developed to observe and cauterize uterine tumors transcervically in a 60-year-old woman. Further major steps in the development of modern hysteroscopy were the introduction of uterine distention with CO_2 and the perfection of quartz light transmission. For a complete description of the development of modern hysteroscopy, the reader is referred to an extensive review by Hamou (9).

Once the hysteroscope had provided clear access to the uterine cavity, the next step was the use of an energy source to destroy the endometrium. Three approaches most recently used include the neodymium:yttrium aluminum garnet (Nd:YAG) laser (10), the urological wire loop resectoscope (11), and the rollerball resectoscope (12).

Patient selection

Indications for endometrial ablation are gradually evolving. They include clinically significant menorrhagia with benign endometrium, failure to respond to standard hormonal therapy, and completion of childbearing. Reports of endometrial ablation have dealt only with patients who have had menorrhagia of significant severity to possibly suggest a hysterectomy. Because amenorrhea cannot be guaranteed, this procedure offers very little advantage to a woman with normal menses who would simply like to avoid further periods. Patients who consider this procedure must be aware that further childbearing cannot be considered. The risk of pregnancy appears to be minimal, although patients cannot be assured that this is a sterilization procedure. The potential for an unpredictable outcome in a subsequent pregnancy, should one occur, must be explained, and sterilization should be offered to appropriate patients. Tubal ligation does not decrease the amount of distending fluid absorbed during the procedure and, therefore, need not be an absolute requirement (13).

The most accurate preoperative investigation is diagnostic hysteroscopy with adequate endometrial sampling. The presence of such intrauterine lesions as polyps, fibroids, or septa might alter the management and is most accurately defined by hysteroscopy and often missed on routine dilatation and curettage (14–16). Patients with atypical endometrium or evidence of neoplasia should not be considered, and those patients with uterine cavities greater than 10 cm in length can expect less than optimal results (17).

Once the determination is made to proceed with surgery, the endometrium is usually rendered atrophic, especially in younger patients, to facilitate ablation and decrease the risk of hemorrhage. This can be carried out using agents that have an antiestrogenic or antigonadotrophic effect.

Recent data suggests that medical preparation may not be necessary, especially in older patients. Suction curettage followed immediately by endometrial ablation, either with the Nd:YAG laser or the resectoscope, resulted in satisfactory decrease in bleeding at six months in 90% of patients in one report (18). Thus, in our practice, we now offer all patients over 40 endometrial ablation with suction curettage without medical preoperative endometrial suppression. This saves money and time for patients and facilitates scheduling the operation.

Techniques

Instrumentation

Safe, successful endometrial ablation requires a light source, viewing system, distending media, and an energy source for the ablation.

Visualization is achieved using a standard light source, fiberoptic cable, and a hysteroscope that is compatible with the operative external sheath required to deliver the attachments for ablation. The use of video, while elegant for teaching purposes, is not an absolute requirement for the performance of the surgery.

Distending media

Intrauterine surgery can only be performed with adequate visualization. The ideal distending medium should be isotonic, nonconductive, clear, electrolytically normal, and, if absorbed, metabolized in the blood stream to nontoxic products. CO_2, while excellent for diagnostic purposes, is not suitable if intrauterine surgery is to be performed.

Glycine is used as a 1.5% solution of the amino acid. It is slightly hypotonic with an osmolarity of 200 mmol/L, essentially nonhemolytic, and electrolyte-free. When absorbed systemically, it is metabolized to serine and glyoxylic acid, which, unfortunately, may cause encephalopathy (19). If it is absorbed, adverse reactions include nausea, vertigo, elevated blood ammonia, and cardiovascular overload (20).

Sorbitol is a 3% solution of D-glycitol, which is a reduced form of dextrose. It is a clear solution that is metabolized to CO_2 and H_2O. It is slightly hypotonic and carries a slight risk of hyperglycemia.

Normal saline and Ringer's lactate are isotonic, crystalloid solutions that are clear and relatively safe if absorbed in moderate amounts. However, because they are conductive, electrosurgical instruments cannot be used. It is popular for use in laser ablation because it is cheap, readily available, and does not solidify when heat is generated by the laser.

Hyskon (Pharmacia, Piscataway, NJ) is a viscous solution of 32%

dextran with a molecular weight of 70,000. It does not contain electrolytes. Its advantages include high viscosity, which effects good uterine distention with small retrograde flow, and its immiscibility with blood, which makes it particularly valuable for diagnostic views with bleeding inside the uterus. However, it has drawbacks, requiring high pressure to achieve irrigation, making evacuation of intrauterine debris difficult. Absorption of small amounts may result in dilutional hyponatremia and pulmonary edema due to the high osmolarity (21). Cases of anaphylaxis (22), adult respiratory distress syndrome, and disseminated intravascular coagulation have also been reported with the intrauterine use of Hyskon (23). Hyskon may also be damaging to instruments if thorough cleansing is not performed immediately after their use.

To obtain satisfactory distention and continuous irrigation, an inflow pressure from 100–110 mmHg is required (24). To achieve this, the solution must be injected either under pressure with a syringe or with a pump or from a bag of solution suspended about 1 m above the patient. Unfortunately, the various methods of distention may lead to intravascular intravasation of fluids unless meticulous monitoring of fluid balance is carried out.

Energy delivery systems

Both lasers and electrical energy can be used to destroy the endometrium. The principles of the equipment for both are the same—an energy generator, an energy delivery system, and an operative sheath for the hysteroscope. The scope must accommodate a lens, an in-flow channel for the distending media, an out-flow channel, and a channel to deliver the energy system for ablation.

Laser energy

The laser used for endometrial ablation is the Nd:YAG. Its advantages include transmission through fine flexible quartz fibers and through liquid distending media and the ability to penetrate tissue to a depth of several millimeters. When the laser beam impacts upon tissue, it is partially absorbed and partially reflected. The amount reflected varies, depending on tissue type and the incident angle of the beam. As the laser energy is absorbed, warming of the tissue occurs and then tissue coagulation. As these changes proceed, the laser energy that is absorbed (forescatter) decreases, and that which is reflected (backscatter) increases. As carbonization of tissue occurs, the amounts of forescatter and backscatter will plateau. This sequence of events is important as energy absorption is decreased as tissue necrosis occurs. The ability of this laser to penetrate through the uterine wall and cause injury is thus restricted, since tissue destruction is limited to a depth of only 4–5 mm.

The quartz fiber used to carry the laser light is bare and consists of a fiber surrounded by a thin plastic covering, beyond which the tip of the fiber extends for a few millimeters. The laser power is generally set

[170]

between 50 and 70 watts. Higher and lower settings may be used under appropriate circumstances. The major disadvantages of the Nd:YAG laser are cost, need for eye filters, and the tedious nature of the ablation when properly and carefully performed.

Electrosurgery

Electrosurgery can be delivered much less expensively. A high-frequency electrosurgical generator is required. One that automatically controls the delivery of both cutting and coagulating currents is optimal. Cutting is achieved by rapidly raising the tissue temperature above 100°C, at which point the cells explode as the intracellular water is transformed to steam. The heat is dissipated in the steam and is not transmitted to the adjacent cells, which will remain intact. Coagulation is achieved by dehydration or deliberate destruction of tissue. For this, the high-frequency current heats the tissue to a temperature less than 100°C, the water is driven out of the cells, and the cytoplasm coagulated. This effect will be obtained by pulsed current. By combining these two currents, the operator can vary the degree of hemostasis, as required during resection.

Due to difficulties in gaining access to the cornual regions of the uterus with the wire loop, a ball-end or rollerball electrode was introduced by Vancaillie to destroy the endometrium thermally by using unipolar cautery as it is rolled along the uterine lining (12). The rollerball has a blunt contact area to dissipate the energy and lessen the probability of perforation, which is a concern when using the hot wire loop. Access to the awkward cornual area is made easier due to the better fit of the rollerball in this fusiform area.

Surgical techniques

Endometrial ablation can be performed with local, general, or regional anesthesia. Once anesthesia has been induced, the patient is placed in the lithotomy position and a Foley catheter is inserted to monitor urinary output. After the usual preparation is made, the cervix is dilated to accommodate the hysteroscope. The sheath is flushed through with the distending medium, and with the fluid running, the hysteroscope and sheath are introduced into the uterine cavity under direct vision. At this point, the technique will differ according to whether laser or electrosurgical energy is used.

Nd:YAG laser

There are three techniques for applying laser energy to the endometrial cavity: stippling, furrowing, and the nontouch technique. Goldrath's original description used the touch technique, which is accomplished by allowing the quartz fiber to be in actual contact with the endometrium during the application of laser energy (10). The endometrium and, presumably, the deeper areas of myometrium are coagulated as the quartz fiber contacts the tissue. If a sapphire tip to the quartz fiber is used, it may limit the depth of destruction, as precision of the cut is not necessary for endometrial ablation.

With the nontouch technique, the fiber is brought as near to the lining of the uterus as possible without touching it. The fiber is also directed as perpendicularly as possible to the uterine wall to decrease the amount of reflection and increase absorption. The endometrium turns white and swells as it is coagulated, but, unfortunately, this change is less clear-cut an endpoint as that in the touch technique. Occasionally, the heat builds up beneath the surface, causing small subendometrial explosions that will detach tissue.

A systematic approach in the uterine cavity is needed to minimize the chances of skipping areas. Unlike the bladder, the uterine cavity is small and it is difficult to apply the laser beam perpendicularly to the lower uterine segments and the sidewalls. Thus, this area is difficult to treat using the nontouch technique. In the touch technique, the fiber can simply be dragged along the wall or used to stipple the walls by gentle pressure. Time required for the procedure ranges from 30 to 120 minutes with the nontouch technique, regarded as the faster method.

The uterus is most efficiently distended when there is a tight fit of the cervix to the hysteroscope. An outflow channel is used to allow bubbles, blood, and debris to be removed from the cavity. Occasional aspiration can be carried out through the outflow channel, where the catheter can be used as necessary to pull out debris.

If the laser is used under direct vision, a special filter is required to protect the operator's eyes. This filter may distort the contrasting colors of the uterine cavity. Preferably, a video camera to display the image on a monitor as a means of retaining color discrimination and protecting operating room personnel's eyes should be used.

Resectoscope

Electrosurgery offers certain advantages for endometrial ablation. It uses known conventionally available equipment that is cheap and familiar to OR personnel. Proper knowledge, selection, and application of electrosurgical energy via the resectoscope is important to perform safe endometrial ablation. Studies have shown that both coagulation and cutting currents applied through the resectoscope wire or ball electrode can produce thermal necrosis as deep as 4 mm (25).

Morphometry of fresh uteri from women undergoing hysterectomy reveals that these uteri can have a myometrial thickness as thin as .4 cm at a distance of .5 cm from the tubal ostia (25). Thus, extreme care must be used with the resectoscope, especially when coagulating or cutting in the uterine horns and upper fundus. In tissues adjacent to a cutting loop, application of electrosurgical current can result in a calculated temperature of up to 5500°C (26). At laparoscopy, thermo couples placed on the surface of the uterus during endometrial ablation have recorded temperature rises as high as 43°C (27). Visual effects on the endometrial surface do not predict actual tissue destruction. Clinically, coagulation current applied slowly at lower powers produces a greater depth of coagulation than cutting current applied at higher powers (28). Thus, we recommend and use cutting current at 100 watts blend one (20% coagulation current) at the fundus and cornu, rapidly and lightly applied, and 75 watts of pure coagulation for the remaining walls of the uterine cavity.

Electrosurgical wire loop resection aims not only to remove the basal layer of endometrium but also the first few millimeters of myometrium, thereby ensuring endometrial destruction. Resection is always started in the fundus and carried down toward the internal os to reduce the risk of uterine perforation. Great care must be taken when using a hot wire loop inside the uterine cavity for endometrial ablation. Laparoscopic control is usually indicated except in the hands of an expert with electrosurgical hysteroscopic ablation. In the hands of an experienced operator, the total operating time can be 20 to 40 minutes.

The strips of resected tissue may be retrieved with periodic curettage or with polyp forceps and saved for histology. At the end of the procedure, the new cavity is inspected, any residual endometrium resected, and any persistent bleeding points coagulated.

Because of difficulties in reaching the cornual area with the wire loop, a ball electrode may be used safely to coagulate the uterine lining without resection. Vancaillie first used the rollerball on the entire uterine cavity as a method of endometrial ablation (12). The ball is rolled along the endometrium under direct vision at a speed of 10–14 mm/sec. The uterine lining is thermally destroyed with a 3–4 mm depth of destruction, which is adequate to reach the basal layer of a thinned endometrium. This technique is easier to master and generally the quickest to perform, with procedure times ranging from 15 to 30 minutes.

All patients undergoing hysteroscopic endometrial ablation should be seen four weeks postoperatively. At that time, uterine sounding can be performed to release any sequestered blood or discharge and to reduce the possibility of developing cervical stenosis.

Results

Nd:YAG endometrial ablation

Since 1981, numerous articles have described procedures with the Nd:YAG laser, documenting follow-up experiences of at least three months and up to six years (Table 14-1). From a total of eight reports, there were 508 patients treated, with 75% becoming amenorrheic or experiencing only slight spotting. A further 68 (14%) continued with regular but light periods, which they considered satisfactory. Only 58 (11%) were considered treatment failures. In the series performed by Davis (33), most failures were attributed to a power setting of 50 watts, and success rates improved considerably when the power was increased to 80 watts. This experience is not shared by others, who report higher success rates at power settings between 25 and 65 watts (34).

The touch technique in the Goldrath series (29) would appear to offer a greater probability of achieving amenorrhea, presumably through the

[173]

Table 14-1 Results of Nd:YAG laser hysteroscopic endometrial ablation

Author	Distending media	Number of patients	Spotting amenorrhea (%)	Satisfactory result (%)	Failure (%)	Complications
Goldrath (29)	Dextrose/ normal saline	216	203 (93%)	3 (1%)	10 (6%)	7 hematometria 1 perforation 1 postop hemorrhage 1 pulmonary edema 1 hyponatremia
Petrucco and Gillespie (30)	Normal saline	24	21 (87%)		3 (13%)	1 perforation 1 bowel injury
Lomano (13)	Normal saline	10	8 (80%)	2 (20%)	0	None
Loffer (17)	Ringer's lactate	33	24 (72%)	7 (21%)	2 (6%)	None
Daniell (31)	Normal saline	144	81 (56%)	41 (28%)	22 (16%)	1 perforation 2 bleeding 1 pulmonary edema
Baggish and Baltoyannis (32)	Hyskon	14	10 (71%)	3 (21%)	1 (7%)	1 pulmonary edema
Davis (33)	Normal saline	25	8 (32%)	5 (20%)	12 (48%)	1 pulmonary edema
Bent and Ostergard (34)	Normal saline	42	27 (64%)	7 (16%)	8 (19%)	3 pulmonary edema
		508	382 (75%)	68 (14%)	58 (11%)	

creation of Asherman's syndrome. The differences in the success rates of recent authors, who were most likely to use a combination of touch and nontouch techniques, suggest the existence of a learning curve for this procedure. Most reports acknowledge that the nontouch technique is quicker to perform. For patients who fail to achieve satisfactory results after one ablation, retreatment is a viable option, with at least a majority reporting acceptable results in one series (35). The presence of fibroids under 12-week size does not seem to be a contraindication to endometrial ablation if menorrhagia is the only symptom and the cavity is not severely distorted. Lomano has reported satisfactory results in 88% of such patients with endometrial ablation using the Nd:YAG laser (36).

Resectoscope resection or ablation

The results with hysteroscopic endometrial ablation (Table 14-2) are similar to those achieved with laser ablation. DeCherney et al. performed total resection in 21 severely ill patients with contraindication to hysterectomy (11). All but one patient who survived her pre-existing disease reported amenorrhea after treatment. Hamou (9) reported his experience with 177 patients, in which some also underwent excision of myomata or polyps during the procedure. All patients underwent partial resection to decrease, but not totally abolish, menstrual flow. Ninety percent (160/177) of patients were satisfied with the result.

A review of eight reports on endometrial ablation with the wire loop resectoscope and/or ball electrode reveals 1,020 patients, treated with 86% satisfied with the results (Table 14-2).

Follow-up of endometrial ablation procedures rarely reveals recur-

[174]

rence of heavy bleeding in patients who initially reported a satisfactory result. Goldrath reported no recurrence of bleeding in patients rendered amenorrheic in follow-up of up to six years (29). Upon repeat hysteroscopy, laser ablation and resection with electrosurgery will show different results. The Nd:YAG ablation leaves a virtually stenotic sealed-down cavity with almost total obliteration of the cavity but no adhesions (32). This is particularly evident in patients treated with the touch technique, which also results in a greater percentage of women becoming amenorrheic. When electroresection is performed, follow-up hysteroscopy reveals only a few adhesions, usually in the cornual regions. The cavity is replaced with a pale, fibrous-looking lining with occasional isolated areas of functioning endometrium, even in patients who report amenorrhea. Repeat hysteroscopy is much easier in those patients who have undergone resectoscope endometrial ablation compared with those with a previous Nd:YAG laser ablation.

Subsequent histological specimens show mainly granulation tissue with no evidence of squamous metaplasia. Interestingly, histological specimens from subsequent hysterectomy due to failed ablation often show adenomyosis (29,38). Although it is unlikely that the presence of adenomyosis will always result in treatment failure, patients with exten-

Table 14-2 Reported results of endometrial ablation with resectoscope

Author	Distending media	Number		Patients with amenorrhea	Patients satisfied	Failure	Complications	Current used
DeCherney et al.[11] (1987)	Hyskon	21	all wire loop excision	18 (86%)	20 (95%)	1 (5%)	None	—
Vancaillie[12] (1989)	Hyskon	14	all ball ablation	10 (67%)	14 (93%)	1 (7%)	None	40–70 watts coagulation
Townsend et al.[37] (1990)	Sorbitol	50	all ball ablation	35 (70%)	45 (90%)	5 (10%)	1 fluid overload hyponatremia	90–100 watts
Maher and Hill[38] (1990)	Glycine	350	part resection part ablation	(95%)	350 (100%)			50 watts coagulation fundus 100 watts cutting sidewalls
Magos et al.[39] (1991)	Glycine	250	all wire loop resection (22 partial only)	105 (42%)	225 (90%)	25 (10%) 16 procedures repeated	4 perforation 1 hemorrhage 2 fluid overload	100–125 watts blended cutting
Hamou[9] (1991)	Glycine	178	all partial resection	0	155 (88%)	22 (12%)	1 perforation 1 hemorrhage 1 bowel injury 2 fluid overload	—
Serden and Brooks[40] (1991)	Glycine	96	all ball ablation	48 (50%)	41 (43%)	8 (7%)	1 fluid overload 1 perforation	—
Daniell et al.[42] (1992)	Glycine	61	all ball ablation	18 (30%)	49 (80%)	12 (20%)	1 perforation in patient with prior Nd:YAG ablation	100 watts blended cutting to fundus 75 watts coagulation to sidewalls
TOTALS		1,020 treated			899 (88%) satisfied			

sive adenomyosis may have a risk of unsatisfactory outcome with persistent or worsening dysmenorrhea.

Most hysteroscopists are now using the resectoscope for endometrial ablation, either with a wire loop or, more commonly, with a rollerball or ball electrodes. Clinical results seem equal, except in the younger patient, where Nd:YAG laser photocoagulation gives a higher amenorrhea rate (41). The resectoscope is easier to learn, quicker to perform, less costly to both patients and operating rooms, and eliminates the need for eye protection during surgery.

Complications

Regardless of the techniques used in endometrial ablation, complications can only be minimized if the surgeon has mastered the skills of operative hysteroscopy. Still, there is some inherent risk in these procedures. The most common complications are hemorrhage, absorption of the distending media, and perforation. Hemorrhage may occur during or after the procedure. The majority of bleeding is seen postoperatively, when the tamponade effect of the pressurized distending media is released and the vessels not fully coagulated will start to bleed. Careful inspection of the uterine cavity after ablation should be undertaken to ensure hemostasis.

The use of distention media under pressure may result in abnormally large volumes being absorbed systemically. Although healthy patients can tolerate several liters of fluid, absorption of a large amount of hypotonic liquid results in a rise in central venous pressure and hyponatremia, which eventually may lead to pulmonary edema (43), water intoxication, or renal damage (44). Isotonic fluids are better tolerated but are also not without risk if enough are absorbed. The use of high viscosity Hyskon has not only been associated with hyponatremia, pulmonary edema, and fluid overload, but also with adult respiratory distress syndrome, disseminated intravascular coagulation, and anaphylaxis if absorbed in significant amounts (45). Fluid overload is invariably associated with prolonged operating time, concomitant surgery, or the use of high distending pressures. Operating room personnel must be trained to carefully monitor fluid use intraoperatively and report it to the surgeon. Logic dictates that extreme caution be practiced in patients with compromised renal or cardiovascular function.

Accidental perforation with the hysteroscope can never be entirely avoided. Special caution should be exercised when using the resectoscope or laser, as the penetrating ability of these instruments is great (46). There is a high risk of organ damage beyond the uterus if perforation occurs. Bowel injury requiring laparotomy has even been reported without uterine perforation while using the rollerball electrode for endometrial ablation (47). Power to the instruments should only be activated when the tip is in clear view and while being drawn back toward the operator.

A recent survey of 4,038 endometrial ablations by the British Society for Gynecologic Endoscopy reported 123 complications (3%), including one death. Most complications (91%) occurred with the wire loop resecto-scope. Uterine perforation occurred most commonly (37%) and most often in cases with inexperienced and/or unsupervised operators (48).

Other complications of hysteroscopic endometrial ablation have been reported or postulated. Goldrath described seven patients with hematometria discovered postoperatively because of cervical stenosis and now recommends routine sounding of the uterus (29). Gas embolism has occurred in two cases of laser ablation, with fatal results (49). This disastrous complication arose from the inappropriate use of a gaseous medium to cool the tip of the fiber during Nd:YAG laser firing. Masking a cancer of the endometrium because of adhesion formation has also been postulated as a long-term complication of endometrial ablation. This is particularly worrisome in patients treated with the Nd:YAG laser, where stenosis may occur and subsequent endometrial bleeding externally may not signal subsequent disease. Although hidden malignancy is unlikely in a population without any previous atypical changes, only long-term follow-up will be able to measure this risk.

It must be remembered that endometrial ablation is not a sterilizing procedure. Patients at risk for pregnancy should be aware of this and possibly offered a concomitant tubal ligation. Reports of pregnancy after endometrial ablation include a term birth by cesarean, delivery with no problems with placental removal (50), and an elective abortion with laparoscopic tubal ligation without complication in a patient who conceived after being amenorrheic for 18 months (51). In our own practice, a patient suffered a spontaneous abortion at three months with severe hemorrhage and secondary retained placenta, which occurred eight months after endometrial ablation. After a first suction curettage, she was transfused and underwent a second operation for hysteroscopy to complete the abortion and remove retained placental fragments and to perform a simultaneous tubal ligation.

Credentialing

Credentialing processes should include the standard three phases of training for any operative endoscopic procedure. These include: (1) obtaining basic privileges for hysteroscopy; (2) after adequate training in hysteroscopy, attending a course that offers hands-on training in the use of the type of energy one wishes to use for endometrial ablation, either laser or electrocautery; and (3) completing a preceptorship with an acknowledged expert in hysteroscopic endometrial ablation.

In our opinion, no one should attempt the procedure until these three steps have been completed. One must obtain some hands-on experience in the operating room, both observing and participating in a case under the direction of an experienced hysteroscopist. Certainly, expertise with the Nd:YAG laser does not imply expertise with the rollerball or wire loop and vice versa. Each technique has subtle differences, and adequate training and hands-on experience is necessary before attempting this procedure on any patient.

[177]

Conclusions

With the advent of the much simpler, less expensive, and rapid technique of electrosurgical endometrial ablation, many surgeons who were discouraged from performing this procedure because of concerns about use of the Nd:YAG will now begin to explore endometrial ablation and offer it to their patients with menorrhagia. There is potential for overuse of the procedure, particularly since it has become simpler to perform with the rollerball electrode. Some physicians and hospitals or free-standing surgery centers are already promoting the procedure with television ads and local media publicity. The goal of all health care providers should be to provide quality health care while minimizing patient costs and risks. Certainly, endometrial ablation in the properly selected and counseled patient meets this goal. It may alleviate a bothersome problem through a simple and rapid outpatient procedure that, if properly performed, can be very safe and effective. As more gynecologists become competent in hysteroscopy and become familiar with these techniques of ablation, there will be an increasing number of women undergoing the procedure. Possibly 25% of the hysterectomies performed in North America today are for menorrhagia only, with benign endometrium and normal cavity. Most of these patients in the next decade could become candidates for a simple outpatient procedure that could replace the more complicated, expensive, and risky hysterectomy. However, proper education of both patients and physicians is critical so that all can benefit from this minimally invasive procedure that offers a cost-effective, simple solution to menorrhagia.

References

1 Dicker RC, Greenspan JR, Strauss LT. Complications of abdominal and vaginal hysterectomy among women of reproductive age in the United States: a collaborative review of sterilization. Am J Obstet Gynecol 1985;144:841–848.

2 Magos AL. Management of menorrhagia. Br J Obstet Gynaecol 1990;300:1537–1538.

3 Asherman JG. Amenorrhea traumatica. Br J Obstet Gynaecol 1948;55:23–30.

4 Asherman JG. Traumatic intrauterine adhesions. Br J Obstet Gynaecol 1950;57:892–895.

5 Phipps JH, Lewis BV, Prior MV, Roberts T. Experimental and clinical studies with radiofrequency-induced thermal ablation for functional menorrhagia. Obstet Gynecol 1990;76:876–881.

6 Ke RW, Taylor PJ. Endometrial ablation to control excessive uterine bleeding. Hum Reprod 1991;6:574–580.

7 Fritsch H. Ein Fall von Volligem Schwund der Gebartmutterhole Nach. Auskratz Centralbl Gynakol 1894;52:52–54.

8 Droegemueller W, Greer B, Makowski E. Cryosurgery in patients with dysfunctional uterine bleeding. Obstet Gynecol 1971;110:467–471.

9 Hamou JE. Hysteroscopy and microcolpohysteroscopy: text and atlas. East Norwalk, Connecticut: Appleton and Lange, 1991:1–12.

10 Goldrath MH, Fuller TA, and Segal S. Laser photovaporization of endometrium for the treatment of menorrhagia. Am J Obstet Gynecol 1981;140:14–19.

11 DeCherney A, Diamond MP, Eavy G, and Polan ML. Endometrial ablation for intractable uterine bleeding: hysteroscopic resection. Obstet Gynecol 1987;70:668–670.

12 Vancaillie TG. Electrocoagulation of the endometrium with the ball-end resectoscope. Obstet Gynecol 1989;74:425–427.

[178]

13 Lomano JM. Photocoagulation of the endometrium with the Nd:YAG laser for the treatment of menorrhagia. J Reprod Med 1986;31:148–150.

14 Brooks PG, Serden SP. Hysteroscopic findings after unsuccessful dilatation and curettage for abnormal uterine bleeding. Am J Obstet Gynecol 1988;158:1354–1357.

15 Gimpelson RJ, Rappold HO. A comparative study between panoramic hysteroscopy with directed biopsies and dilatation and curettage. Am J Obstet Gynecol 1988;158:489–492.

16 Loffer FD. Hysteroscopy with selective endometrial sampling compared with D&C for abnormal uterine bleeding: the value of a negative hysteroscopic view. Obstet Gynecol 1989;73:16–21.

17 Loffer FD. Hysteroscopic endometrial ablation with the Nd:YAG laser using a nontouch technique. Obstet Gynecol 1987;69:679–682.

18 Lefler HT, Sullivan GH, Hulka JF. Modified endometrial ablation: electrocoagulation with vasopressin and suction curettage preparation. Obstet Gynecol 1991;77:949–953.

19 Hoekstra PT, Kahnoski R, McCarnish MA. Transurethral resection syndrome—a new perspective: encephalopathy with associated hyperammonemia. J Urol 1983;130:740–747.

20 Madsen PO, Madsen RE. Clinical and experimental evaluation of different irrigating fluids for transurethral surgery. Invest Urol 1965;3:122–130.

21 Leake JF, Murphy AA, Zacur HA. Noncardiogenic pulmonary edema: a complication of operative hysteroscopy. Fertil Steril 1987;48:497–499.

22 Knudtson ML, Taylor PJ. Uberempfindlichkeitsreaktion auf dextran 70 (Hyskon) wahrend einer hysteroskopie. Geburtshilfe Frauenheilkd 1976;36:263–264.

23 Jedeikin R, Olsfanger D, Kessler I. Disseminated intravascular coagulopathy and adult respiratory distress syndrome. Life-threatening complication of hysteroscopy. Am J Obstet Gynecol 1990;162:44–45.

24 Magos AL, Lockwood GM, Baumann R, Turnbull AC, Kay JDS. Correspondence: absorption of irrigating solution during transcervical resection of the endometrium. Br Med J 1990;300:1079–1084.

25 Duffy S, Reid PC, Smith JHF, Sharp F. In vitro studies of uterine electrosurgery. Obstet Gynecol 1991;78:213–220.

26 Honig WM. The mechanism of cutting in electrosurgery. IEEE Trans Biomed Eng 1975;22:58–62.

27 Indman PD, Brown WW. Uterine surface temperature changes caused by electrosurgical endometrial coagulation. J Reprod Med 1992;37:667–670.

28 Indman PD, Soderstrom RM. Depth of endometrial coagulation with the urologic resectoscope. J Reprod Med 1990;35:633–635.

29 Goldrath MH. Hysteroscopic laser surgery. In: Baggish MS, ed. Basic and advanced laser surgery in gynecology. Norwalk, Connecticut: Appleton-Century-Crofts, 1985:357–372.

30 Petrucco OM, Gillespie A. The neodymium:YAG laser and the resectoscope for the treatment of menorrhagia. Med J Aust 1991;154:518–520.

31 Daniell JF. Endometrial ablation. In: Azziz R, Murphy AA, eds. Practical gynecologic endoscopic pelvic reconstruction. New York: Springer-Verlag, 1991:173–181.

32 Baggish MS, Baltoyannis P. New techniques for laser ablation of the endometrium in high-risk patients. Am J Obstet Gynecol 1988;159:287–292.

33 Davis JA. Hysteroscopic endometrial ablation with the neodymium-YAG laser. Br J Obstet Gynaecol 1989;96:928–932.

34 Bent AE, Ostergard DR. Endometrial ablation with the neodymium-YAG laser. Obstet Gynecol 1990;75:923–925.

35 Gimpelson RJ, Kaigh J. Endometrial ablation repeat procedures. J Reprod Med 1992;37:629–634.

36 Lomano J. Endometrial ablation for the treatment of menorrhagia: a comparison of patients with normal, enlarged, and fibroid uteri. Laser Surg Med 1991;11:8–12.

37 Townsend DE, Richart RM, Paskowitz RA, Woolfork RE. Rollerball coagulation of the endometrium. Obstet Gynecol 1990;76:310–313.

38 Maher PJ, Hill DJ. Transcervical endometrial resection for abnormal uterine bleeding. Aust NZ Obstet Gynaecol 1990;30:357–360.

39 Magos AL, Baumann R, Lockwood GM, Turnbull AC. Experience with the first 250 endometrial resections for menorrhagia. Lancet 1991;337:1074–1078.

40 Serden SP, Brooks PG. Treatment of abnormal uterine bleeding with the gynecologic resectoscope. J Reprod Med 1991;36:697–699.

41 Daniell JF, Kurtz BR, Ke RW. Hysteroscopic endometrial ablation using the rollerball electrode. Obstet Gynecol 1992;80:329–332.

42 Magos AL, Baumann R, Turnbull AC. Transcervical resection of endometrium in women with menorrhagia. BMJ 1989;298:1209–1212.

43 Feinberg BI, Gimpelson RI, Godier RN. Pulmonary edema after photocoagulation of the endometrium with the Nd:YAG laser: a case report. J Reprod Med 1989;34:431–434.

44 Morrison LMM, Davis J, Sumner D. Absorption of irrigating fluid during laser photocoagulation of the endometrium in the treatment of menorrhagia. Br J Obstet Gynaecol 1989;96:346–352.

45 Mangar D, Gerson JI, Constatine RM, Lenzi V. Pulmonary edema and coagulopathy due to Hyskon (32% Dextran-70) administration. Anesth Analg 1989;68:686–687.

46 Perry CP, Daniell JF, Gimpelson RJ. Bowel injury from Nd:YAG endometrial ablation. J Gynecol Surg 1990;6:199–203.

47 Kivnick S, Kanter MH. Bowel injury from rollerball ablation of the endometrium. Obstet Gynecol 1992;79:833–835.

48 Macdonald R, Phipps J, Singer A. Endometrial ablation: a safe procedure. Gynaecol Endosc 1992;1:7–9.

49 Baggish MS, Daniell JF. Castastrophic injury secondary to the use of coaxial gas-cooled fibers and artificial sapphire tips for intrauterine surgery: a report of five cases. Laser Surg Med 1989;9:581–584.

50 Hill DJ, Maher PJ. Pregnancy following endometrial ablation: a case review. Gynaecol Endosc 1992;1:47–49.

51 Mongelli JM, Evans AJ. Pregnancy after transcervical endometrial resection. (Letter to the Editor). Lancet 1991;338:110.

15 Gonadotropin-Releasing Hormone (GnRH) Analog Therapy—Uterine Leiomyoma

ESTHER EISENBERG

Excessive blood loss is one of the major surgical risks associated with hysterectomy or myomectomy (1). At times, blood transfusion may be required. Many factors correlate with the necessity for blood transfusion, including the preoperative hemoglobin, uterine size, and the skill of the surgical team. Morevoer, myomectomy or hysterectomy may be more difficult to accomplish when multiple myomas distort the normal anatomic landmarks of the uterus and the pelvis. This situation may result in excessive operative time and anesthetic exposure, which is associated with an increased incidence of infection and other surgical morbidity.

Gonadotropin-releasing hormone (GnRH) agonist analogs have been introduced into the pharmacologic armamentarium, enabling the surgeon to affect the preoperative hemoglobin and, to some extent, uterine size. These agents should be considered prior to surgery in all patients with uterine myomas as preoperative adjuncts, just as preoperative iron therapy or preoperative autologous blood collection is often recommended as a means to reduce surgical risks. Not all patients will be candidates for GnRH analog therapy, but the following discussion will delineate the pharmacology, physiology, rationale, risks, and benefits of GnRH therapy so that an informed recommendation may be offered.

Background

The discovery and synthesis of GnRH in 1971 by two independent laboratories of Guillemin and Schally (2), the elucidation of the physiologic actions of GnRH by Knobil and colleagues (3), and the development of long-acting GnRH analogs has made possible a new era of therapeutic intervention (4).

GnRH is a decapeptide (Figure 15-1) produced in the arcuate nucleus of the medial basal hypothalamus. It is secreted in a pulsatile fashion, which is critical for the pituitary synthesis and secretion of follicle stimulating hormone (FSH) and lutenizing hormone (LH). GnRH pulses normally occur at approximately hourly intervals. Native GnRH is rapidly degraded in the pituitary by endopeptidases and, consequently, has a very short half-life of four to eight minutes.

The physiologic imperative of pulsatile GnRH secretion for the establishment and maintenance of menstrual cyclicity (5) is the basis for the

[181]

Figure 15-1 Amino acid sequence of native GnRH agonist analogs often have modifications at positions 6 and 10.

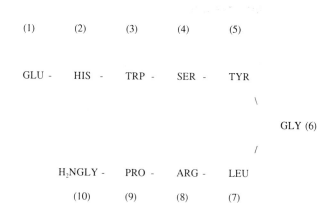

application of long-acting GnRH agonists. Knobil and colleagues demonstrated that continuous exposure of the pituitary gonadotrope to GnRH leads to an initial increase and then a rapid decline of FSH and LH secretion. This observation provided clinicians a means to "shut down" the pituitary. The decline in gonadotropin secretion occurs because of *down-regulation,* a decrease in the number of unoccupied GnRH receptors, and *desensitization,* an inability of the GnRH receptor complex to initiate the normal intracellular events necessary for hormone synthesis and release (6). This eventually leads to the cessation of ovarian steroidogenesis and the development of a hypoestrogenic state (a reversible medical oophorectomy).

GnRH agonists are synthetic analogs of native GnRH with amino acid substitutions most commonly at position 6 and/or 10, which stabilize the structure of the peptide and make it less susceptible to enzymatic degradation (Figure 15-1). In contrast to native GnRH, which has a very short half-life, the synthetic agonist analogs have a much longer half-life (80 minutes to six hours) because of increased GnRH receptor binding affinity and decreased degradation in the pituitary (7).

When the pituitary is exposed to a synthetic GnRH agonist, initially a brief period of increased release of FSH and LH (~ one to three weeks) occurs, followed by a prolonged decrease in FSH and LH secretion and resultant inhibition of ovarian steroidogenesis. In practice, then, the use of a GnRH agonist results in inhibition of pituitary FSH and LH release, similar to the state that occurs during continuous exposure to native GnRH. One major advantage of the agonist analogs is that the inhibition of steroidogenesis can be achieved by administration of a daily subcutaneous injection, monthly depot, or twice daily nasal spray rather than by continuous infusion because these analogs have a longer half-life and increased potency as compared to native GnRH (Table 15-1).

GnRH *antagonists* are synthetic analogs of GnRH that competitively inhibit GnRH binding to its receptor complex but do not stimulate intracellular events necessary for synthesis and release of the gonadotropins. Theoretically, the GnRH antagonists have the advantage of immediately inhibiting FSH and LH release, thus more rapidly inhibiting ovarian steroidogenesis without an initial stimulatory effect (8).

Presently, however, the GnRH *agonist* analogs are more useful clinically than the antagonists because of the propensity of the currently

Table 15-1 GnRH agonists available for clinical usage

GnRH agonist	Trade name	Administration	Dosage/ Frequency	Half-life
Leuprolide acetate	Lupron	Subcutaneous injection -or-	1 mg (0.2 ml) daily	3 hr
		Depot IM injection	3.75–7.5 mg monthly	
Nafarelin acetate	Synarel	Nasal spray	1–2 200 mg spray in alternate nostrils twice daily	4.3 hr
Goserelin acetate	Zoladex	Subcutaneous depot	3.6 mg every 28 days	6 hr
Histrelin acetate	Supprelin	Subcutaneous	10 µg/kg/day	

available GnRH antagonists to elicit histamine release, which is not well tolerated by patients.

Rationale

Uterine leiomyomata occur in approximately one out of four women over 30 years of age. Of these women, 20–50% have symptomatic uterine fibroids requiring treatment (9). Pelvic pressure, pelvic pain, abdominal discomfort, urinary urgency or frequency, back pain, and difficulty with bowel movements are symptoms directly related to the mass and location of the fibroids pushing or exerting pressure on adjacent pelvic structures.

Symptomatic excessive or prolonged uterine bleeding often leading to iron deficiency anemia is related to the uterus's inability to adequately contract the spiral arterioles of the endometrium and to the increased surface area of the endometrium secondary to the enlarged uterine mass. Treatment options include surgery for symptomatic myomata, watchful waiting, and, in selected cases, hormonal therapy.

Surgery, either hysterectomy or myomectomy, is the most effective treatment modality in symptomatic women; however, it is fraught with increased risks of bleeding, adhesion formation, and surgical difficulty when the uterus is enlarged or distorted. The procedure of choice depends on the patient's age, her desire for fertility, her desire to retain her uterus, and the extent of her symptoms. Myomectomy is indicated in women who have solitary pedunculated fibroids, infertility, or recurrent pregnancy loss secondary to myoma, wish to maintain their childbearing potential, are unsure of their future reproductive desires, or who, for personal reasons, wish to retain their uterus. Hysterectomy is indicated in those women who have completed childbearing, have recurrent myomata, have significant surgical risk factors in whom elimination of the possibility of recurrence is desirable, or who want definitive therapy.

Specific factors that have an impact on the ease of the surgery (be it myomectomy or hysterectomy) and on intraoperative blood loss include

[183]

Table 15-2 GnRH agonist preoperative therapy

Advantages
• Control of acute symptoms of pain and bleeding
• Restoration of hemodynamic stability
• Provides time to donate autologous blood
• Timing of surgery becomes semielective rather than emergent
• Decreases intraoperative blood loss in larger uteri
• Facilitates hysteroscopic myomectomy
• Reduces surgical risks

the size of the uterus; number, size, and location of the myoma(s); and ease of removal of the myoma from the uterine site.

Since uterine leiomyomata are hormone-sensitive tumors containing identifiable estrogen and progesterone (10,11) and GnRH (12) receptors, various hormonal regimens have been employed either as attempts at definitive medical therapy or preoperatively in an attempt to shrink uterine myomas. High-dose progestin therapy has been attempted based on the rationale that progestins inhibit estrogen's actions at the cellular level (13). Although degenerative changes in myomas exposed to large doses of progestins have been reported, most uterine myomas respond poorly to progestins. Danazol, an impeded androgen that inhibits ovarian steroidogenesis and blocks the production of estradiol by aromatase inhibition also has been used to shrink uterine myomata with varied results. Maximal shrinkage of 20–25% has been observed following the use of Danazol 800 mg daily for three months (14).

GnRH agonists have been utilized since 1983 as adjunctive preoperative therapy for myomectomy or hysterectomy because of their excellent suppression of ovarian steroidogenesis (15,16). In patients with excessive uterine bleeding related to myomata, GnRH agonists more rapidly suppress ovarian estrogen production than either progestagens or Danazol and are much more effective in controlling hemorrhage.

In several studies, GnRH agonists have been shown to reduce uterine volume 34–61% (17,18,19,20). Individual myomata have a more varied response ranging from 0% to 100% reduction in size within six months of therapy. Maximal reduction of uterine size generally occurs within three months of therapy.

A concomitant beneficial effect usually observed within one month of GnRH agonist therapy is the relief of pelvic symptoms because of the

Table 15-3 GnRH agonist therapy

Side effects
• Insomnia
• Headaches
• Amenorrhea
• Vaginal dryness
• Decreased libido
• Vasomotor symptoms/Hot flashes
• Reversible decreases in bone density

decrease in uterine size. Amenorrhea during therapy is the rule, with an occasional exception. During this therapeutic window, iron therapy may be instituted in anemic women to restore hemoglobin concentration to normal. In addition, autologous blood may be collected and stored for possible perioperative use. In women with intermittent uterine bleeding that continues during therapy, several possible explanations may be considered. These include infrequent or inappropriate self-administration (more likely to occur with subcutaneous or nasal routes as opposed to depot), an extraneous source of estrogens (ovarian tumor), or unrecognized uterine leiomyosarcoma.

The use of a GnRH agonist as adjunctive therapy is effective in reducing intraoperative blood loss both during myomectomy and hysterectomy. Most likely, the reduction in intraoperative blood loss is due to a decrease in uterine blood flow during therapy and the shrinkage of the uterus and the myomata, making the surgery technically less difficult.

Potentially, the greatest advantage of GnRH agonist adjunctive therapy is in the patient with submucous leiomyomata (21). Prior to the advent of hysteroscopy, treatment of submucous leiomyomata required laparotomy, with entry into the endometrial cavity for myomectomy and subsequent recommendation for cesarean section as the preferred mode of delivery. The ability to perform hysteroscopic resection of submucous leiomyoma enables these to be successfully removed transvaginally in 75–80% of cases. The addition of GnRH agonist pretherapy reduces the operative time, intraoperative bleeding, volume of infused medium utilized, and failure rate to 3% in patients treated with GnRH agonist for three months prior to hysteroscopy.

Other hormonal means of manipulating uterine leiomyomata may be on the horizon. Although still experimental, the regression of uterine leiomyomas in response to the antiprogesterone RU486 (22) has been reported to be comparable to that observed with GnRH agonists. Successful reduction in leiomyoma size has also been accomplished with the administration of the GnRH antagonist, Nal-glu GnRH (50 mg/kg/day) (23). A 50% reduction in uterine leiomyoma volume was observed after four weeks of therapy. The major therapeutic advantage of the GnRH antagonist over the agonist analogs is that shrinkage of uterine volume occurs more rapidly because of the absence of the initial stimulatory effects that commonly occur during GnRH agonist therapy.

Common to all the hormone manipulations of uterine leiomyomas is their transient effects. Most studies have shown a return to pretreatment uterine and leiomyoma volumes within six months after discontinuation of therapy with GnRH agonist or GnRH antagonist. This finding has prompted consideration of prolonged continuous GnRH agonist administration with concomitant add-back hormonal therapy (24) as an alternative to surgery. In a pilot study carried out for two years (25), five premenopausal women with uterine myomas were treated for three months with GnRH agonist with resultant 40–50% shrinkage. This was followed by GnRH agonist plus low-dose estrogen and progestin hormone replacement for an additional 24 months. No significant regrowth of the myomas or bone loss was measured, and the side effect of hot

[185]

flashes was prevented. However, a prospective, randomized, double-blind, placebo-controlled crossover trial in 16 women, evaluating the effects of leuprolide acetate (1 mg/sc/day) compared to simultaneous administration of leuprolide acetate (1 mg/sc/day) and medroxyprogesterone acetate (20 mg/day), revealed that when both hormones are administered simultaneously, a reduction in uterine volumes does not occur (26). If the medroxyprogesterone acetate is "added back" after three months of treatment with GnRH agonist, there is an initial reduction followed by modest increase in uterine volume to approximately 80% of pretreatment levels.

The data on add-back regimes is still evolving; however, unless there is a serious prohibition to surgery, the majority of women will most likely opt for definitive surgical therapy (either myomectomy with a recurrence risk of 10–30% or hysterectomy) rather than be maintained on continuous prolonged medical therapy. When weighing advantages and disadvantages of prolonged therapy, costs and inconvenience of ongoing medical therapy should be discussed.

Advantages

When is it appropriate to use GnRH analogs?

GnRH analog therapy facilitates the management of uterine leiomyomata by enabling the gynecologist/surgeon and patient to exert some control over a potentially explosive clinical situation. If the patient is experiencing acute symptoms of pain or excessive bleeding, then administration of a GnRH analog will result in a rapid reduction of pain and pressure effects (uterine shrinkage) as well as rapid onset of amenorrhea (cessation of ovarian steroidogenesis), often within two to three days. Although medical therapy is a temporizing measure, it permits the scheduling of definitive surgery at a time convenient for both the patient and the physician.

In addition, preoperative analog treatment enables the physician to institute oral iron therapy to correct iron deficiency anemia, if present, and allows the patient to bank autologous blood without further growth of the myoma, should blood transfusion be necessary perioperatively.

Moreover, because of the 40–50% shrinkage in uterine size and the reduction in uterine blood flow attendant with GnRH analog therapy, there will be the associated benefits of decreased intraoperative blood loss, especially in pretreatment uteri estimated to be greater than 16 weeks' gestational size. Myomectomy may be more easily accomplished, perhaps through a smaller uterine incision, potentially resulting in a reduced area for adhesion formation. In some instances, utilization of a GnRH prior to surgery will facilitate performance of a myomectomy in a situation where hysterectomy would have been necessary.

Finally, pretreatment with GnRH analog significantly increases the success of hysteroscopic resection of submucous leiomyomata while reducing intraoperative blood loss and operative time. All these benefits may be observed within three months of agonist therapy and one month of antagonist therapy. GnRH analogs are not appropriate in postmenopausal women in the presence of abnormal uterine bleeding of unknown etiology, when the uterine myoma is extensively calcified, or when a leiomyosarcoma is suspected because of rapid growth (27).

Side effects

The major side effects of the GnRH agonist analogs are related to the hypoestrogenic state attained. These include hot flashes in the majority of women, occasional irregular spotting or sparse vaginal bleeding, and, less frequently, headaches, vaginal dryness, and loss of libido. Because the contribution of this period of hypostrogenism to the eventual development of osteoporosis is a concern, GnRH agonists are not recommended for long-term (>6 months) use. Recent investigations have explored the feasibility of concomitant add-back therapy, either with estrogen or medroxyprogesterone acetate as potential ways to avert the development of osteoporosis. The results have been favorable for estrogen add-back but less favorable for medroxyprogesterone acetate (see above).

Summary

A rationale for the use of GnRH analogs has been presented. As with all treatment modalities, the decision to use a GnRH analog preoperatively must be individualized to meet a specific patient's needs and desires. One of the major advantages of the GnRH analogs as adjunctive therapy for myomectomy or hysterectomy is that these agents enable the physician to shift acutely symptomatic myomas from an emergent to a semielective medical condition. This provides the time necessary to orchestrate a successful outcome for the patient and the physician.

References

1 Wiskind AK, Thompson JD. Abdominal myomectomy: reducing the risk of hemorrhage. Sem Repro Endoc 1992;10:358–365.
2 Schally AV. Aspects of hypothalamic regulation of the pituitary gland. Science 1978;202:18–28.
3 Knobil E. The neuroendocrine control of the menstrual cycle. Rec Prog Hormon Res 1980;36:53–88.
4 Karten MJ, Rivier JE. Gonadotropin-releasing hormone analog design structure-function studies toward the development of agonists and antagonists: rationale and perspective. Endocrine Rev 1986;7:44–66.
5 Belchetz PE, Plant TM, Nakai Y, et al. Hypophyseal responses to continuous and intermittent delivery of hypothalamic gonadotropin-releasing hormone. Science 1978;202:631–634.
6 Conn PM. The molecular basis of gonadotropin-releasing hormone action. Endocrine Rev 1986;7:44–66.
7 Handelsman DJ, Swerdloff RS. Pharmacokinetics of gonadotropin-releasing hormone and its analogs. Endocrine Rev 1986;7:95–105.
8 Vickery BH. Comparison of the potential for therapeutic utilities with gonadotropin-releasing hormone agonists and antagonists. Endocrine Rev 1986;7:115–124.

9 Wallach EE. Myomectomy. In: Thompson JD, Rock JA, eds. Te Linde's operative gynecology. 7th ed. Philadelphia: JB Lippincott 1992:647–662.

10 Pollow K, Geilfuss J, Boguoi E, Pollow B. Estrogen and progesterone binding protein in normal human myometrium and leiomyoma tissue. J Clin Chem Clin Biochem 1978;16:503–511.

11 Soules MR, McGarty KS Jr. Leiomyomata: steroid receptor content variation with normal menstrual cycle. Am J Obstet Gynecol 1982;135:6–11.

12 Wiznitzer A, Marbach M, Hazum E, et al. Gonadotropin-releasing hormone specific binding sites in uterine leiomyomata. Biochem Biophys Res Commun. 152:1326–1331.

13 Whitehead MI, Townsend PT, Pryse-Deuren J, et al. Effect of estrogen and progestins on the biochemistry and morphology of the postmenopausal endometrium. N Engl J Med 1981;305:1599–1603.

14 Maheux R, Lemay A. Uterine leiomyoma: treatment with GnRH agonist. In: Rolland R, Chadha DR, Williamson WNP, eds. Gonadotropin down regulation in gynecologic practice. New York: Alan R. Liss, 1986:297–311.

15 Friedman AJ. GnRH agonist therapy for uterine leiomyomata. In: Barbreri RL, Friedman AJ, eds. Gonadotropin-releasing hormone analog. New York: Elsevier 1991:39–61.

16 Adamson GD. Treatment of uterine fibroids: current findings with gonadotropin-releasing hormone agonists. Am J Obstet Gynecol 1992;166:746–751.

17 Maheux R, Gulloteau C, Lemay A, et al. Luteinizing hormone-releasing hormone agonist and uterine leiomyoma: a pilot study. Am J Obstet Gynecol 1985;152:1034–1038.

18 Filicori M, Hall DA, Loughlin JS, et al. A conservative approach to the management of uterine leiomyoma: pituitary desensitization by a luteinizing hormone-releasing hormone analogue. Am J Obstet Gynecol 1983;147:726–727.

19 West CP, Lumsden MA, Laursen S, et al. Shrinkage of uterine fibroids during therapy with goserelin (Zoladex): a luteinizing hormone-releasing hormone agonist administered as a monthly subcutaneous depot. Fertil Steril 1987;48:45–51.

20 Friedman AJ, Rein MS, Harrison-Atlas P, et al. A randomized, placebo-controlled, double-blind study evaluating leuprolide acetate depot treatment before myomectomy. Fertil Steril 1989;52:728–733.

21 Perino A, Chianchiano N, Petronio M, Cittadini E. Role of leuprolide acetate depot in hysteroscopic surgery: a controlled study. Fertil Steril 1993;59:307–510.

22 Murphy AA, Kellel LM, Morales AJ, Roberts VJ, Yen SSC. Regression of uterine leiomyomata in response to the antiprogesterone RU486. J Clin Endocrinol Metab 1993;76:513–517.

23 Kettel LM, Murphy AA, Morales AJ, et al. Rapid regression of uterine leiomyomas in response to daily administration of gonadotropin-releasing hormone antagonist. Fertil Steril 1993;60:642–646.

24 Friedman AJ, Lobel SM, Rein MS, Barbieri RL. Efficacy and safety considerations in women with uterine leiomyomas treated with gonadotropin-releasing hormone agonists: the estrogen threshold hypothesis. Am J Obstet Gynecol 1990;163:1114–1119.

25 Friedman AJ. Treatment of leiomyomata uteri with short-term leuprolide followed by leuprolide plus estrogen-progestin hormone replacement therapy for two years: a pilot study. Fertil Steril 1989;51:526–528.

26 Carr BR, Marshburn PD, Weatherall PT, et al. An evaluation of the effect of gonadotropin-releasing hormone analogs and medroxyprogesterone acetate on uterine leiomyomata volume by magnetic resonance imaging: a prospective randomized double-blind placebo-controlled, crossover trial. J Clin Endocrinol Metab 1993;76:1217–1223.

27 Smith S, Cooper M, Schinfeld JS. Incidental finding of endolymphatic stromal myosis during luteinizing hormone-releasing hormone agonist therapy for suspected benign uterine myomata. J Reprod Med 1992;37:980–982.

16 Hormonal Management of Dysfunctional Uterine Bleeding

JOEL T. HARGROVE

Definition

Uterine bleeding is a common condition for which reproductive-aged women seek gynecologic care. Such bleeding may be too frequent, excessive in duration or amount, or occur at an unexpected time. As a diagnostic entity, *dysfunctional uterine bleeding* refers to bleeding that does not result from a systemic or reproductive tract pathologic process. Because it is a diagnosis of exclusion, serious disorders presenting with vaginal bleeding must be ruled out before embarking on a therapeutic course. In most cases, dysfunctional uterine bleeding results from anovulatory cycles. Some authorities include as a subgroup the bleeding that occurs with ovulation or with corpus luteum defects; however, most consider the derangements associated with anovulation as the best explanation of dysfunctional uterine bleeding. The American College of Obstetricians and Gynecologists suggests that the term "anovulatory uterine bleeding" may be preferable to "dysfunctional uterine bleeding" (1).

Although dysfunctional uterine bleeding may occur at any time during the reproductive years, it is especially common at the beginning of menstrual life and during the transition phase preceding the menopause. When anatomic and pregnancy-related problems are excluded, hormonal and medical therapy are almost always successful in controlling the bleeding problem, and surgical intervention should rarely be required (2).

The normal menstrual cycle

Evaluation and treatment of abnormal cycle bleeding requires an understanding of the normal ovulatory cycle. Because there is individual variation in the parameters that define a "normal menstrual cycle," groups of individuals have been used to average these parameters, so, in reality, we are speaking of an "average menstrual cycle" (3). In Vollman's comprehensive review on the temporal aspects of the menstrual cycle, he credits the first attempt at defining the normal menstrual cycle to Mary Putnam Jacobi in 1876, when she published her observations on the fluctuations of the basal body temperature (4). Since that time, the menstrual cycle has been the subject of extensive investigation (3,5).

Menarche occurs at an average age of 12.8 years in American girls (6). After ovulatory cycles are established, most will range from 25 to 30 days in length; however, the ovulatory cycle length is variable and can range from 21 to 36 days (3). The usual duration of menstrual flow is four to six days, with an average blood loss of 30 ml. When bleeding is more than 80 ml, iron deficiency anemia may result (7). In the decade preceding the menopause, variations in ovarian function result in a shortening of the menstrual cycle length by two to three days (8,9). The menopause usually occurs around age 50 years (10).

The hallmark of menstruation is the bloody endometrial effluent from the uterus. While menstrual bleeding defines both the beginning and the end of an ovulatory cycle, menstruation signifies the failure of the previous ovulation to culminate in the establishment of pregnancy. By the time menstrual bleeding is detected, neuroendocrine and ovarian events are already initiating a new cycle and another attempt at reproduction. Failure of the corpus luteum to maintain progesterone secretion allows pituitary follicle-stimulating hormone to rise and a new cohort of follicles are recruited to play their role in the succeeding cycle.

The human endometrium is a dynamic tissue that undergoes cyclic periods of cellular proliferation and differentiation in response to a changing ovarian hormone environment during the menstrual cycle (Figure 16-1). The endometrium, which lines the uterine cavity, consists of epithelial glands surrounded by a vascular-rich connective tissue stroma. Distinct histologic and cytologic changes can be appreciated within the endometrium at each stage of the menstrual cycle (11). In the preovulatory phase of the cycle, estradiol dominates the endocrine milieu that results in the rapid proliferation and thickening of the endometrium (Figure 16-2). Most structural changes in the endometrium are the result of estrogen stimulation. Following ovulation, the human corpus luteum continues to secrete estradiol, but progesterone is the principle product of the postovulatory ovary. Under the dominant influence of progester-

Figure 16-1 Ovarian hormone control of the endometrium.

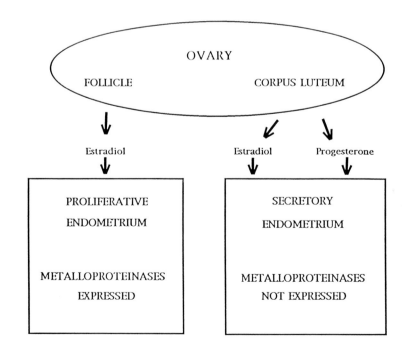

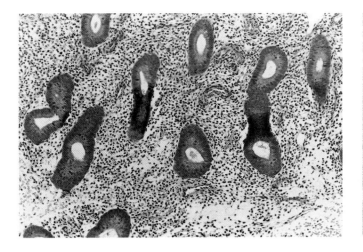

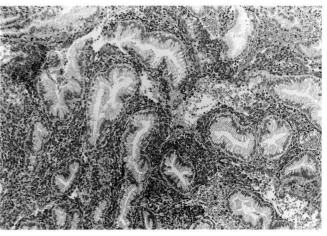

Figure 16-2 Proliferative endometrium (courtesy of Dr. Harold W. Ferrell).

Figure 16-3 Secretory endometrium (courtesy of Dr. Harold W. Ferrell).

one, cellular differentiation results in a secretory endometrium (Figure 16-3). Specific receptors for estradiol and progesterone are present in the endometrium, and the expression of these receptors is regulated by the action of these steroids. The expression pattern of steroid receptors within different endometrial cell types as well as the concentrations of these receptors varies considerably during the course of the cycle. Estradiol receptor levels peak during the late proliferative stage of the cycle, while progesterone receptors are highest during the early luteal phase (12,13). Additionally, endometrial cells elaborate local paracrine hormones, such as growth factors, in response to steroid stimulation. Together, ovarian steroids and local growth factors may act to control the cyclic expression of many proteins within the endometrium. An example of such proteins are matrix metalloproteinases of the stromelysin family, which appear to be necessary for tissue remodeling during endometrial growth (14–16). Interestingly, endometrial metalloproteinase expression is suppressed by progesterone, and these enzymes appear to play a major role during the breakdown of endometrial tissue at menstruation. While supportive data does not yet exist, it is tempting to speculate that steroid-dependent production or suppression of endometrial metalloproteinases may play an important role in the etiology of dysfunctional uterine bleeding.

If pregnancy fails to occur, the corpus luteum involutes, luteal estrogen and progesterone production declines, endometrial steroid receptors decrease, the endometrium loses its hormonal support, and menstruation follows (Figure 16-4). Normal menstruation results from progesterone withdrawal, and continued support with estrogen alone will not postpone the withdrawal bleeding; however, progesterone will delay bleeding. In anovulatory cycles, bleeding eventually occurs from estrogen withdrawal, and this bleeding can be postponed by the administration of progesterone. Therefore, progesterone is essential to controlling uterine bleeding from an estrogen-primed endometrium (17).

These cyclic events occur at approximately monthly intervals from

[191]

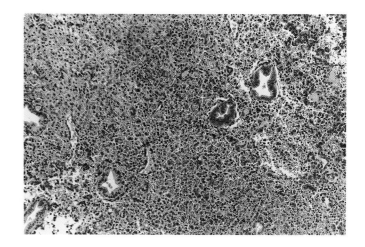

Figure 16-4 Menstrual phase endometrium (courtesy of Dr. Harold W. Ferrell).

puberty until the menopause unless interrupted by pregnancy, hormonal imbalance, failure to ovulate, or pathologic processes.

Diagnosis

As with most disorders encountered in clinical medicine, the success of the therapy depends on the accuracy of the diagnosis. A careful history and physical examination, when combined with selective laboratory, imaging, and biopsy data, will establish the diagnosis in most cases. Dysfunctional uterine bleeding is a product of anovulation and, by definition, is not caused by pregnancy abnormalities or pathologic processes, local or systemic, involving the reproductive tract. These processes should be excluded to arrive at an accurate diagnosis. Accidents of pregnancy can be ruled out by history, pelvic examination, measurement of serum β-hCG, and selective use of ultrasound.

Ovulatory cycle bleeding

Characteristically, regular ovulatory cycles frequently exhibit some degree of premenstrual molimina and dysmenorrhea. Bleeding occasionally occurs at ovulation in the absence of anatomic lesions. Ovulation bleeding presents with regular bleeding occurring every two weeks and is rarely excessive. Basal body temperature will confirm the diagnosis. This bleeding is usually self-limiting and only requires observation in most cases.

Intermenstrual bleeding or heavy, prolonged menstrual bleeding during ovulatory cycles may result from anatomic lesions and be confused with dysfunctional uterine bleeding. Coagulopathies associated with platelet disorders or deficient clotting factors, such as von Willebrand's disease or leukemia, may cause intermenstrual bleeding and heavy bleeding at menstruation in ovulatory cycles. These disorders are usually encountered in the early postmenarcheal years. Past history, family history, and hematologic evaluation are important in establishing the diagnosis (18).

Because of the potential life-threatening implications, bleeding resulting from genital organ malignancies must be excluded. They tend to occur in the later reproductive age years. Lesions involving the vulva, vagina, and cervix are usually visible or palpable on careful examination. The diagnosis can be confirmed by biopsy. Endometrial cancer should be suspected when there is a history of chronic anovulation such as occurs with polycystic ovarian disease. Transvaginal ultrasonography may be helpful, but the diagnosis must be established by endometrial biopsy or dilatation and curettage.

Ovarian malignancies can cause bleeding problems by interfering with normal ovarian function. These lesions are notorious for escaping early diagnosis. Careful attention must be given to a history of vague abdominal pain. A family history of ovarian cancer is important and, if positive, warrants a measurement of serum CA-125 level. Careful pelvic exam for ovarian enlargement should be done. Transvaginal sonography can be a valuable aid in detection, and color Doppler studies may be helpful in evaluating the malignant potential of ovarian masses.

A number of benign genital tract conditions may result in vaginal bleeding and need to be excluded. Such entities as vaginal or cervical polyps and leiomyomas are usually obvious at pelvic examination. Infectious processes involving the vagina, cervix, and uterus and foreign bodies, such as a retained tampon or intrauterine device, may occasionally be the etiology of the bleeding. The presence of iron deficiency is more likely to be associated with an organic lesion causing the bleeding (19). Endometriosis can be suspected by the history of pain, bleeding, and infertility. Vaginal spotting in the late luteal phase three to five days before full menstrual flow is typical of endometriosis. Palpable tender nodules are helpful but can easily be missed. Laparoscopy may be necessary to confirm the diagnosis.

Anovulatory bleeding

Anovulation is central to the mechanism of dysfunctional uterine bleeding (Figure 16-5). Anovulation in a premenopausal woman results in unopposed estrogen stimulation to the endometrium and eventually to

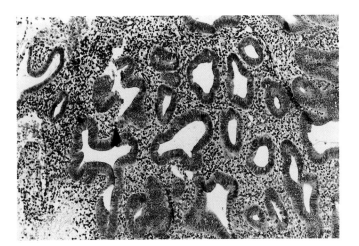

Figure 16-5 Anovulatory endometrium showing persistent estrogen effect (courtesy of Dr. Harold W. Ferrell).

estrogen withdrawal bleeding. Unopposed estrogen may also result in bleeding when cellular proliferation exceeds the ability of the endometrium to maintain its integrity. Because of the decreased production of prostaglandin $F_{2\alpha}$ in this situation, the bleeding is usually less painful (20). The amount of flow depends on the degree and duration of estrogen stimulation to which the endometrium has been subjected.

Anovulatory cycles and bleeding are common around menarche and at the menopause. Anovulatory cycles that result in bleeding or amenorrhea are sometimes associated with aerobic exercise programs, endocrine disorders such as prolactinoma, hyperthyroidism, hypothyroidism, Cushing's syndrome, and congenital adrenal hyperplasia, or drug therapy.

In many patients, chronic anovulation or oligo-ovulation is suggested by irregular cycles and periods of amenorrhea that have been present since menarche. Because of the prolonged unopposed estrogen stimulation in such patients, endometrial biopsy should be done to rule out hyperplasia or cancer.

Laboratory studies, biopsies, and vaginal sonography

A complete blood count is central to the evaluation of bleeding. History and physical examination should guide the selection of laboratory tests. If the process is chronic, suction endometrial biopsy can be done with relatively little pain with one of the small disposable suction curettes, such as the Pipelle (Unimar, Wilton, CT) (21–23). This procedure can be done during the examination and provides a tissue sample that correlates well with that obtained at formal dilatation and curettage. Some lesions, such as endometrial polyps and submucous leiomyoma, are cryptic but can be revealed by transvaginal sonography with saline injected for contrast (Figure 16-6).

Treatment

The initial treatment will depend on the duration and severity of the bleeding and should be directed to controlling the acute bleeding. Although rare, hypovolemic shock, if present, requires stabilizing the patient with appropriate fluid and blood replacement and dilatation and curettage to control the hemorrhage. The majority of patients do not present with this catastrophic picture, and the acute bleeding can be controlled by hormonal therapy with one of the progestational agents. Treatment of dysfunctional uterine bleeding with these compounds is rational and successful (24). Norethindrone acetate 5 mg or medroxyprogesterone acetate 10 mg given three times daily will nearly always be successful in controlling the bleeding. The duration of this regimen depends on the hematologic status of the patient. If no anemia is present, the progestin may be stopped after 10 to 12 days and withdrawal bleeding will occur. In those patients with anemia, the progestin regimen is continued until the anemia is sufficiently corrected to safely allow withdrawal bleeding. Depending on the individual patient, usually three to six weeks will be satisfactory.

[194]

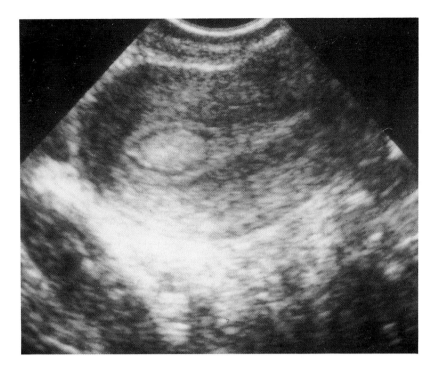

Figure 16-6 Endometrial polyp found to be the cause of persistent bleeding. Transvaginal ultrasound view with real-time injection of normal saline into the uterine cavity.

After an acute bleeding incident is controlled, the management goal of dysfunctional uterine bleeding is to avoid repeated bleeding episodes and prevent the long-term sequelae of anovulation, endometrial hyperplasia, and cancer (25). Therapy that meets these goals is progestational agents. The reproductive desire of the patient needs to be considered in choosing the source of the progesterone. If pregnancy is the issue, ovulation induction would be the treatment of choice. If contraception is needed, birth control pills should be considered. If contraception is not an issue, cyclic administration of norethindrone acetate 2.5 to 5 mg or medroxyprogesterone acetate 5 to 10 mg 10 to 14 days of each month will establish regular cycles. About 30% of the patients will develop significant premenstrual syndrome symptoms (depression, bloating, etc.) on these agents. To some extent, these symptoms are dose-related and may be helped by giving the smaller dose of progestin for a shorter time each cycle. For example, norethindrone acetate 2.5 mg may be given the 16th through the 25th day of each cycle.

Natural progesterone can be used in those cases where other progestins are unacceptable. Progesterone, 100 mg in oil, can be given intramuscularly once monthly. This is somewhat cumbersome due to the need for an injection and the tendency for pain at the injection site. Progesterone suppositories 50 mg used vaginally or rectally for 10 to 14 days of each month work well; however, some individuals object to the discharge that tends to accompany this therapy.

Progesterone, when micronized and suspended in an oil carrier, can reach therapeutic levels when given orally (26). Progesterone has a short half-life and must be taken in multiple dosages, usually two or three times daily with a total dose of at least 300 mg to consistently achieve a secretory endometrium (27). Dosages at this level will frequently cause intolerable drowsiness due to the 5α metabolites of progesterone (28).

In summary, dysfunctional uterine bleeding is associated with anovulation and can be successfully managed in most women by cyclic administration of progestin. The progestin can be given alone or as a part of a combination therapy with estrogen in one of the various birth control pills.

References

1 American College of Obstetricians and Gynecologists. Dysfunctional uterine bleeding. Technical Bulletin no 134. Washington DC: American College of Obstetricians and Gynecologists, October 1989.

2 Speroff L, Glass RH, Kase NG. Dysfunctional uterine bleeding. In: Clinical gynecologic endocrinology and infertility. Baltimore: Williams & Wilkins, 1989:265–282.

3 Abraham GE. The normal menstrual cycle. In: Givens JR, ed. Endocrine causes of menstrual disorders. Chicago: Year Book Medical Publishers, Inc., 1978:15–44.

4 Vollman RF. The menstrual cycle. Major problems in obstetrics and gynecology, Vol 7. Philadelphia: WB Saunders, 1977.

5 Southam AL, Gonzaga FP. Systemic changes during the menstrual cycle. Am J Obstet Gynecol 1965;91:142–165.

6 Zacharias L, Rand WM, Wurtman RJ. A prospective study of sexual development and growth in American girls: the statistics of menarche. Obstet Gynecol Survey 1976;31:325–337.

7 Hallberg L, Hogdahl AM, Nilsson L, Rybo G. Menstrual blood loss: a population study. Acta Obstet Gynecol Scand 1966;45:320–351.

8 Treloar AE, Boynton RE, Behn BG, Brown BW. Variation of the human menstrual cycle through reproductive life. Int J Fertil 1967;12:77–126.

9 Sherman BM, Korenman SG. Hormonal characteristics of the human menstrual cycle throughout reproductive life. J Clin Invest 1975;55:699–706.

10 Krailo MD, Pike MC. Estimation of the distribution of age at natural menopause from prevalence data. Am J Epidemiol 1983;117:356–361.

11 Noyes RW, Hertig AT, Rock J. Dating the endometrial biopsy. Fertil Steril 1950;1:3–25.

12 Lessey BA, Killam AP, Metzger DA, Haney AF, Greene GL, McCarty KS Jr. Immunohistochemical analysis of human uterine estrogen and progesterone receptors throughout the menstrual cycle. J Clin Endocrinol Metab 1988;67:334–340.

13 Healy DL, Hodgen GD. The endocrinology of human endometrium. Obstet Gynecol Survey 1983;38:509–529.

14 Nelson KG, Takahashi T, Bossert NL, Walmer DK, McLachlan JA. Epidermal growth factor replaces estrogen in the stimulation of female genital tract growth and differentiation. Proc Natl Acad Sci USA 1991;88:21–25.

15 Bell SC, Jackson JA, Ashmore J, Zhu HH, Tseng L. Regulation of insulin-like growth factor-binding protein-1 synthesis and secretion by progestin and relaxin in long-term cultures of human endometrial stromal cells. J Clin Endocrinol Metab 1991;72:1014–1024.

16 Rodgers WH, Osteen KG, Matrisian LM, Navre M, Giudice LC, Gorstein F. Expression and localization of matrilysin, a matrix metalloproteinase, in human endometrium during the reproductive cycle. Am J Obstet Gynecol 1993;168:253–260.

17 Greenblatt RB, Karpas AE. Dysfunctional uterine bleeding. In: Givens JR, ed. Endocrine causes of menstrual disorders. Chicago: Year Book Medical Publishers, Inc., 1978:249–263.

18 Wentz AC. Abnormal uterine bleeding. In: Jones HW III, Wentz AC, Burnett LS, eds. Novak's textbook of gynecology. Baltimore: Williams & Wilkins, 1988:378–396.

19 Vercellini P, Vendola N, Ragni G, Trespidi L, Oldani S, Crosignani PG. Abnormal uterine bleeding associated with iron-deficiency anemia. Etiology and role of hysteroscopy. J Reprod Med 1993;38:502–504.

20 Carr BR. Disorders of the ovary and female reproductive tract. In: Wilson JD, Foster DW, eds. Williams textbook of endocrinology. Philadelphia: WB Saunders, 1992:733–798.

21 Hill GA, Herbert CM, Parker RA, Wentz AC. Comparison of late luteal phase endometrial biopsies using the Novak curette or Pipelle endometrial suction curette. Obstet Gynecol 1989;73:443–445.

22 Fothergill DJ, Brown VA, Hill AS. Histological sampling of the endometrium—a comparison between formal curettage and the Pipelle sampler. Br J Obstet Gynaecol 1992;99:779–780.

23 Stovall TG, Ling FW, Morgan PL. A prospective, randomized comparison of the Pipelle endometrial sampling device with the Novak curette. Am J Obstet Gynecol 1991;165:1287–1290.

24 Yen SSC. Chronic anovulation caused by peripheral endocrine disorders. In: Yen SSC, Jaffe RB, eds. Reproductive endocrinology. Philadephia: WB Saunders, 1991:576–630.

25 Bayer SR, DeCherney AH. Clinical manifestations and treatment of dysfunctional uterine bleeding. JAMA 1993;269:1823–1828.

26 Hargrove JT, Maxson WS, Wentz AC. Absorption of oral progesterone is influenced by vehicle and particle size. Am J Obstet Gynecol 1989;161:949–951.

27 Lane G, Siddle NC, Ryder TA, Pryse-Davies J, King RJ, Whitehead MI. Dose-dependent effects of oral progesterone on the oestrogenised postmenopausal endo-metrium. Br Med J [Clin Res] 1983;287:1241–1245.

28 Arafat ES, Hargrove JT, Maxson WS, Desiderio DM, Wentz AC, Andersen RN. Sedative and hypnotic effects of oral administration of micronized progesterone may be mediated through its metabolites. Am J Obstet Gynecol 1988;159:1203–1209.

INDEX